TITANIA'S

Aroma Magic

TITANIA'S

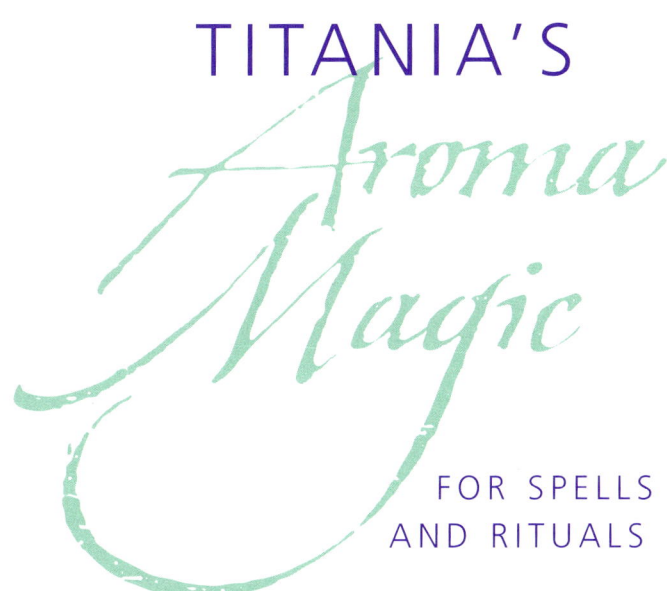

Aroma Magic

FOR SPELLS AND RITUALS

TITANIA HARDIE

ILLUSTRATED BY TRINA DALZIEL

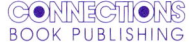

CONNECTIONS
BOOK PUBLISHING

This book is dedicated to all the scent-loving souls who will enjoy it and spread their
fragrant magic in a delicious web right across the world to cheer us all

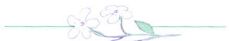

A CONNECTIONS EDITION
This edition published in Great Britain in 2004 by
Connections Book Publishing Limited
St Chad's House, 148 King's Cross Road
London WC1X 9DH
www.connections-publishing.com

British Library Cataloguing-in-Publication data available on request.

ISBN 1-85906-160-5

1   3   5   7   9   10   8   6   4   2

Phototypeset in Weiss, Fruitiger and La Figura using QuarkXPress on Apple Macintosh
Origination by Chroma Graphics (Overseas) PTE Ltd, Singapore
Printed and bound by Hung Hing Offset Printing Co. Ltd, China

Contents

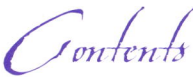

Introduction

Wisteria flowers twisting around a bedroom window; lemon trees blooming in the summer; sweet, damp earth on a crisp spring day with a gentle breeze; home-baking in the house of our childhood; freshly laundered linen; the perfume of our favourite female relative … Scent transports us, it seems, to every lovely place that we have ever been. In a direct path to the memory, the smells that bring us face to face with our past persuade our brains that time stands still, and that unicorns (to echo Shakespeare!) are still possible. Scent is so evocative – smell, perhaps, the most emotional of all our senses. It is the knowledge of this potent fact that drives fragrance houses to spend millions selecting the right balance of aromas; they are selling us love – or the hope to be more confidently loved – in beguilingly beautiful bottles.

This book of magical rituals associated with scent embraces the same concept. We exude the most subtle of scents when we are happy, sexy, sad, vulnerable, comfortable, which animals understand instinctively. And when we are in love, we give off specific chemical signals that include almost imperceptible scents. When we borrow the fragrance of a beautiful flower, we are borrowing its erotic language to entice someone closer to us. And if we know which scents, and which rituals, will help us exude everything from confidence to happiness and sensuality, our lives are enhanced in the simplest and most direct way.

Thus, I am beginning this book – and writing these words – on a perfect, very early English spring day, with a bouquet of highly scented narcissi (jonquils) on my desk. To speak to you or write without the bliss of some exotic aroma would be unjust. My senses are stirred, and our journey through olfactory heaven will be honest and shared. Bring your heightened awareness with you, and let us discover the magic of scent. We will look at the different ways to harness scent, and learn more about the language we use to select specific single note fragrances, or groups of scents, in oils and candles, posies of fresh herbs and flower-filled vases.

Aromatic oils can literally change our lives, by making our homes more welcoming, our workspace more enticing and satisfying to work in, our private rooms more romantic, and our inner selves more inspired. And when we join this to simple rituals, practised by our ancestors for generations, to put our minds in the most positive frame, we have a powerful magical aura. So select your favourite scent, or room spray, or pluck a bloom of your choice as your companion while you read on. The path we tread will be fragrant and uplifting, and you will be making magical things happen to you. Breathe in deeply, and relax …

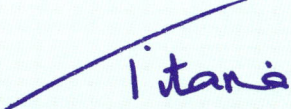

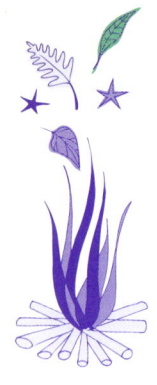

CHAPTER ONE

Aroma Power

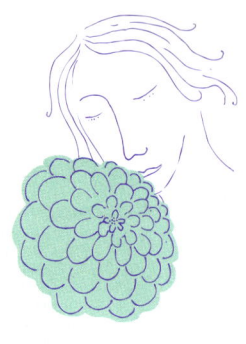

In this first chapter we will explore the history of the use of oils and scent
in rituals, from incense and woods to distillations of flowers and herbs.
What are essential oils? And how do they affect our minds? We will consider the
way in which scent contributes to our consciousness, and how it affects our self-control
and self-motivation. This highlights other connections between the mind and its ability to
trigger healing, happiness and assertiveness. Scent can play a significant part in these
positive states, and makes a direct connection through the olfactory bulb with our brain.
But we also respond individually to aroma in groups – woods, florals, herbs, resins,
fruits and so on – and this response can help us to understand our own personality
in terms of scent. Find out how you respond to scent, and the aromas that your
personality is drawn to will be your best tools for creating magic
and success around you!

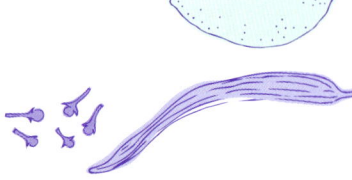

The Rise of Aromatic Magic

Long ago our ancestors discovered the power of aroma. Whether it was through burning leaves in camp fires or using a variety of the woods that were available, they must have understood the impact of particular scents on the mood of the tribes or clans: juniper, frankincense and olive wood all have an uplifting effect when burned; pine and citrus woods invigorate us and give us courage. Indeed, the word 'perfume' recognizes the release of scent *par fume* – through smoke. This was the first form of incense, and smouldering leaves and herbs were used to cleanse, purify and sanctify an area for religious rituals from the beginnings of time. Tellingly, scented smoke is common to all religions and cultures across the world.

Try burning scented leaves on an open fire or when you barbecue.
In the summer, meats skewered on to herbed stems, like rosemary, infuse the food
with flavour and bestow aromatic bliss on the garden!

Herbs and flowers create an aromatic rainbow for our senses. While the colour and shape pleases the eye, it is the gift of scent that so uplifts humanity. When we colour our environment with great bowls of aromatic herbs or fragrant seasonal blooms, we also fill the air with intoxicating smells that are literally a balm to our senses. Depending on the choice of scent, our mood can be light and bubbly, more earthy and sensuous, calm and focused, or even energized and daring. Scent is strangely invisible to us, but is as tangible as silken fabrics and soft breezes. It might be a metaphor for the world we cannot see, a seductive link between mind, body and spirit, between the world of physical reality and the world of our dreams. All tastes are not the same, but aroma can be released into the atmosphere like musical notes to evoke a range of emotions in all of us.

Our entire system of smell is complex in its workings and yet direct in its relationship with our brain, and thus with our feelings and moods. One part of our olfactory system is in the nose, with the other right inside the brain: the olfactory bulb is actually the top of the nose, between the brow bones, and is part of the brain itself. This means that messages received through smell are instant, fresh and immediate in contrast to our other senses, which are filtered through our nerves and passed along to the brain by a relay system. One quick inhalation of lavender or roses may instantly transport us to our past – to a favourite aunt or a wonderful, enchanted old house. Our emotions respond deeply and quickly to memories stirred through smell.

How do we detect smell?

Much research is still being done to understand the numerous ways in which we pick up aromas, and the revitalized interest in aromatherapy is contributing to a desire for this knowledge, but we have at least learned that our organ of smell is very sensitive and sophisticated. While we only differentiate four different types of taste – sweet, salt, sour, bitter – we may perceive as many as ten thousand different types of smell. When we inhale through our noses, we come into contact with the molecules that are released from aromatic substances. This is how vital information used originally for our protection and survival as a species was obtained: smelling smoke, food, or other predators on the wind was a means of finding food or escaping dangers. Being able to distinguish subtle differences between herbs and flowers might have meant the differentiation between a toxic or non-toxic variety. The scent that enters our brains is stored in the memory, which we retain for decades, it seems, and even across generations. Fresh citrus blooms may delight the child of someone born in the Mediterranean, for instance, although they have little or no experience of the actual plant themselves; perhaps the scent stirs an inherited memory.

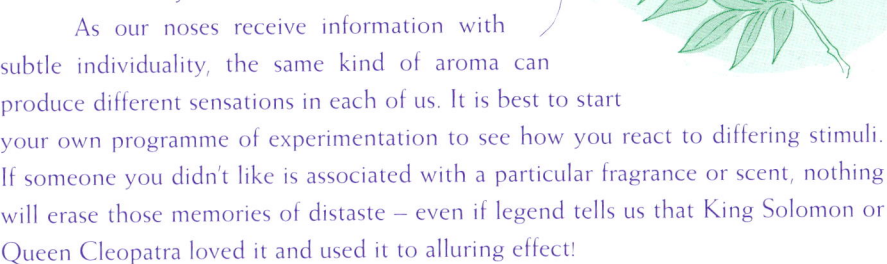

As our noses receive information with subtle individuality, the same kind of aroma can produce different sensations in each of us. It is best to start your own programme of experimentation to see how you react to differing stimuli. If someone you didn't like is associated with a particular fragrance or scent, nothing will erase those memories of distaste – even if legend tells us that King Solomon or Queen Cleopatra loved it and used it to alluring effect!

Essential oils and magic

Apart from commercial perfumes, the most accessible way of experimenting and using scent is with essential oils, which are now so widely available that the olfactory journey is both exciting and affordable. An essential oil can be extracted from flowers, leaves, stems, barks and even seeds; and if a flower or herb has a scent, there will be an oil 'essence' somewhere. All of these oils are antibacterial, and some also have other properties, but their function includes the task of attracting pollination and putting pests off their trail. Perhaps they even contribute to the way a plant 'talks' to other plants, or conveys its 'soul': I certainly think that this is a possibility.

And this brings us to magic. To make magic work, your mind must be strong and focused. You can succeed at the most extraordinary tasks – manifest and make actual the most astonishing of wishes – if you can successfully fix your sights on a goal and draw it to you. Chemical signals can be borrowed from various sources, such as colour, sound and taste, but there is nothing more potent to use with your magic than aroma. The chemical signals from the plant kingdom speak through the ether, with more eloquence than we can attempt. In a way, we are harnessing the energies of many items when we work ritual, whether coloured ribbons and fabrics or the souls of little plants and flowers. Scent is the chief ambassador: it goes forth to the upper planes, and asks that our wishes be bestowed properly. It also persuades our inner psyche to behave in concert with our goals: it makes us bolder, more confident, more exotic, so that we too can exude exactly the right body language in the appropriate situation to attract what we are seeking.

So this is an invitation to explore scents of different types and to understand the different ways to utilize them: publicly, when others are in your company; privately, when you are using them to heighten your mind and react with the language of your personal being; and in everyday situations, freely and easily, to effect the results you hope for in life. It starts, I believe, with finding out more about your 'scented self', looking at how you respond to smells of different families, and discovering which aromas work for you. This brings us to the question of your 'scent personality', and whether it is fixed or open to growth and change, and how it can be discovered through your feelings about aroma.

The Aromatic Soul Personalities

Our personalities are an enigma. Within the same families, with shared cultural conditioning and similar genetic information, we are still individual in our ideas, understanding, emotions, responses. To make magic work for, and to weave a mystical harmony between, ourselves in our own identity and the world in which we live, it is enlightening to understand something about our personal reactions, how we see ourselves, how (perhaps) others might see us, and how we respond to different aromas. Our personality influences the way we express ourselves to the outside world. People make cursory judgements by such aspects of our character and taste as they can detect. And perfumes work hard to persuade us which 'soul' we aspire to be, and to offer us our wish in a scented aura!

Glamorous? Sensuous? Educated? Strong? Old-fashioned? Scent helps you express all of these facets of your being. Earthy? Passionate? Enigmatic? Serene? Once you identify your dominant temperament and characteristics, it is easy to select the aromas that help you exude everything you would wish.

Which soul are you?

Read the following table to identify the soul you feel most strongly akin to. We are seldom simple enough to be neatly boxed into any one group, so don't be surprised if you have aspects of more than one. You may love citrus smells and be more bubbly and outgoing when you are in holiday mood in the warmer months, and become more attracted to roses and lilies when you feel romantic or nostalgic, but you can still be a woody-scented soul, desiring cedarwood or sandalwood when you are in private. Try to identify the group or groups that most strongly seem to say your name!

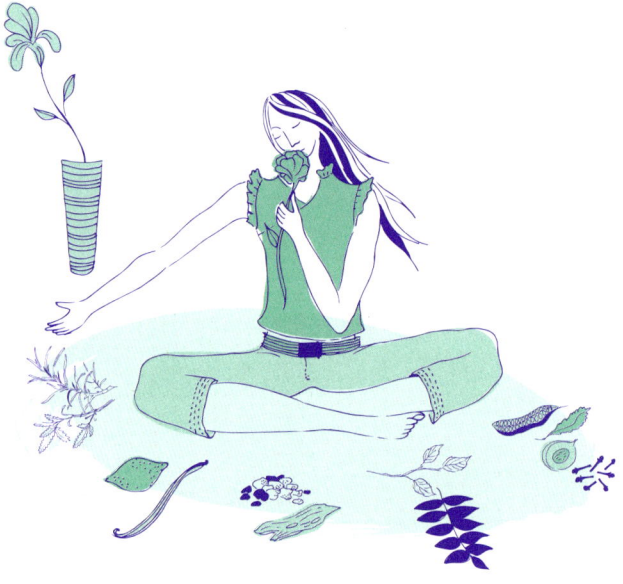

THE HERB SOUL

Herb oils and scents, such as:
basil, hyssop, lavender (leaves), lemon balm,
lovage, marjoram, mint, rose geranium,
rosemary, sage, thyme

If you feel empathy with these scents,
you are likely to be:
kind-hearted, generous to others, reliable,
helpful to friends, honest, sympathetic,
emotional and curious. You are practical
and good with your hands.

Home body or party animal?
Home body! You are a good nurturer, good
gardener and may work from home.

Traits to guard against?
You are very demanding, need to be
appreciated desperately, and when dejected
or under pressure you can be a martyr.

THE FLOWER SOUL

Flower oils and scents:
camomile, carnation, gardenia, hyacinth,
jasmine, lavender flower, lemon and lime
blossom (not the full fruit smell), lily, linden
flower, mimosa, narcissus, neroli, peony,
rose, tuberose, violet, wattle

If you respond emotionally to these scents
you are probably:
artistic, charismatic, emotionally vivid, sexy,
idealistic, a perfectionist, fashionable, peace-
loving. You have real flair and originality,
and take time over your appearance.

Home body or party animal?
Party animal, for sure! You are flirtatious,
desirable and like to be admired and noticed.
You are a good host, but can be quite
competitive.

Traits to guard against?
You can think too much of appearance, be
snobby, interfere in others' lives, and rely
on sex rather than love!

THE FRUIT SOUL

*Oils are taken from the fruits of the plant,
not the flowers:*
apricot, avocado, bergamot, all citrus fruits
(lemon, lime, orange, mandarin, grapefruit),
clove, hops, juniper, vanilla

*If you respond imaginatively to this group,
you are probably:*
loyal, dependable, friendly, vibrant, sanguine,
easy-going, intuitive, hard-working,
intelligent, good with people, true to yourself,
a good organizer and love to get behind
a cause or interest.

Home body or party animal?
A bit of both. You like birds-of-a-feather
friends, keeping them for years and
entertaining them without fuss frequently.
And you love your home.

Traits to guard against?
You are too indecisive, impatient with slower
people, self-critical and critical of others when
you're depressed; also prone to work burnout.

THE WOOD AND BARK SOUL

*This group covers oils distilled from trees and
wood, including resins:*
the balsams, benzoin, camphor, cedarwood,
frankincense, galbanham, myrrh, pine,
rosewood, sandalwood

If you come alive to these scents, you may be:
brave, clever, earthy, grounded, focused,
perspicacious, wise, fair-minded, principled,
persevering, truthful, charitable, intellectual,
up-to-date, well read, a 'doer'

Home body or party animal?
A public-minded person, you have a private
life in an ordered home, but are away from
home often. Good in both arenas.

Traits to guard against?
Sometimes you can be moody, controlling
of other people, bored with under-achievers
and hard-hearted!

THE LEAF SOUL

This is scent distilled from leaves:
bay, birch, clover, eucalyptus, myrtle,
patchouli, petitgrain, pine, tea tree

If you respond to these scents, you are:
quiet, considered, creative, self-improving,
drawn to books, an interesting speaker,
calming, peace-loving

Home body or party animal?
Home body, but welcoming to friends.
You will have a good library and a
comfortable relaxing space.

Traits to guard against?
Becoming paranoid, feeling 'got at',
and worrying too much.

THE SPICE SOUL

These are extracted from several parts of spice plants:
anise, aniseed, caraway, cinnamon, clove,
coriander, cumin, fennel, galangal, ginger,
mace, nutmeg, peppers, saffron

If you are drawn primarily to these, you are:
joyful, animated, energetic, outgoing,
confident, humorous, entertaining, restless,
bubbly, a high-flyer

Home body or party animal?
Parties: you make even a coffee break a social
event! You love people, fascinate them, give
a lot and are an original party-giver.

Traits to guard against?
A lover of too much luxury, you can be a
show-off and often don't listen to others.

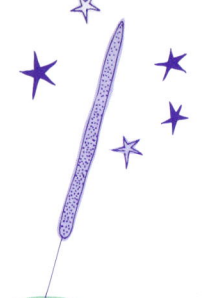

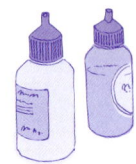

CHAPTER TWO

Everyday Magic

Now we know something more about our responses to smell,
and have thought about our feelings for different groups of aromas,
we are ready to consider ways of putting magic – through aroma – into our
ordinary day, on a regular basis. Sometimes we can do this just by adding scent
to our routine, such as diffusing oils to improve our mind-set in the office, at home
or on social occasions, or spritzing room spray when we are feeling flat or tired or
finding it hard to concentrate. But here, too, I hope you will find some interesting
new ways to make magical things happen by introducing delightful aromas into
unexpected places. Think of the appropriate aroma by considering its effect and
remember the groups that work best and brightest on your own psyche,
which we explored at the end of the first chapter.
And then, let us start weaving some scented
magic into our lives …

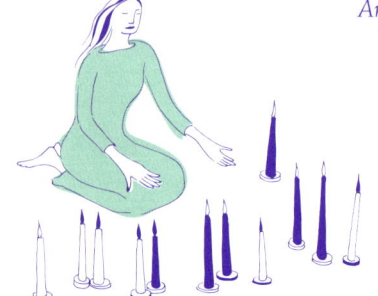

Scented Choices

The brain is processing smells continually. We pick up the aromatic molecules in the cilia of receptor cells in the nose, and the messages are then transmitted to the olfactory bulb at the top of the nose, near the brow. This scent is quickly translated into enzyme response: the smell of bread baking, for instance, transmits a signal to make us feel hungry. Aroma can almost produce a self-hypnotic state: certainly, it can contribute to one. A focused mind, which emits an aura of control, confidence and energy, can make things happen, introducing positive 'tensions' into a flat atmosphere. There are always results from such a spark! With this in mind, each of us has the capacity to make a little bit of magic every day, in common situations, with pleasing results.

The limbic system, the zone that is most affected by smell, is the seat of our emotions and psychological impulses. When we *smell*, we *feel*. The two routes to this emotional response are through *olfaction* (smell) and *absorption* (through the skin). So, scent released via incense, diffusers and candles has a direct impact on the limbic system, while the effect from massage or bathing has a double effect, with the oils being absorbed through the skin as the warmth simultaneously releases the scent to the nose.

We need to understand something of the differences between the aromatic groups to exploit their best potential for us in spells and rituals. Rituals, for example, frequently ask that we anoint our brow, wrists or other parts of our body with oils, or even that we bathe before an important rite. This utilizes both methods of focusing the brain: absorption and olfaction. Spells are more likely to require us to release the aromas to the nose, which is simpler and demands less preparation. This is highly effective for most spells, as the scent quickly bolsters our emotions and our moods to fit the task.

Candles

For working 'everyday' magic – that is, to make magical things happen regularly in commonplace situations – it is helpful to understand why certain aromatic choices are better than others. A scented candle encourages intimacy. If you are working alone in a fairly small area, the use of a scented candle will be perfect for stimulating or focusing your moods and energies, and allow you to inject creative, magical thoughts into everyday tasks. It is also a perfect choice for bedroom or bathroom, dinner table or living room, because the magical effect of the scent works in tandem with the play of light from the flame and the chosen colour of the candle itself. Warm pinks with floral notes make an atmosphere more playful and loving; reds impregnated with spicy aromas raise our pulse to fuel our passions; herbal yellows can alert the brain to boost our intellect; leafy greens – such as birch and pine – can help us recover our fatigued health; blues added to many scents, like geranium, lavender and camomile, calm us after a long day.

Your diffuser

If the area you are working in is bigger, however, then diffusion of the pure essential oil has a broader impact. If you can get colleagues to acquiesce, it is also wonderful used in an office, where you can weave a spell of magic and good humour over colleagues and, at the same time, refresh everyone with an aromatic blast that will ease over-tired minds and invigorate the brain cells. This is what I call being the 'witch in the boardroom' and everyone will love you for it!

In a mentally challenging day, then, aromatic magic released directly from the essential oils will lift the soul and clear the mind – literally, like a breath of fresh air. This can increase your creativity and help you to concentrate more effectively. Your memory can be made more potent and your attentiveness more tangible. This in turn attracts respect from others and a feeling of prowess in your work – a kind of magic in which luck plays no part!

However, in magic-making and in Wiccan ideology, there is a belief in the special quality and spiritual resonance released by the plants themselves through their essences: it is rather like accepting the view that a tree has a powerful and majestic persona of its own, which is worth respecting and harmonizing with. As such, the power of the scent to enchant the senses is taken slightly further, as we are also harnessing the energies and essences of the plants to our benefit. This takes us beyond the simple understanding that aromatic oils will deodorize or sanitize a room and into an understanding that they also impart a sense of light and positivity – a lightness of being, sharing their souls with us and making us cheerful.

Green herbaceous aromas, such as thyme, rosemary or bergamot, have a slightly sharp fragrance that stimulates clarity and professionalism; basil and rosemary effectively provoke our powers of memory, and can also be used emblematically in magical spells to evoke a positive feeling about memories and people in our past. Sweeter fragrances have an aromatic power of a different kind: lavender and lemon scents bid a welcome to guests and lovers; woody oils encourage inner warmth and a celebratory feeling when our spirits are otherwise plunged into wintry realms; and romantic encounters are anticipated by rose, orange blossom and geranium, while gardenia and jasmine invite deeper passions!

Incense

Incense can be used for ritualistic purposes – perhaps when you have a special occasion and wish to make the space special or when you have guests. Smoke itself is so ceremonial. Few people I know are not transported to another time, another place, when they sniff the delicious high-church perfumes that might be associated with childhood or solemn occasions. Some scents, like frankincense, make us feel 'nobler of the mind'; some, like benzoin, encourage spiritual and altruistic emotions. Incense is available in such a variety of shapes, textures and scents, that it is no longer a 'sixties time warp' to waft it around the home. Do so when you are clearing away an argument, moving house or getting over the end of something in your life – an old job or the loss of a relative, perhaps.

But let us consider some cheerful ways to use scent with the purposes of making magic each day, in a very informal and relaxed fashion. Never miss an opportunity to take a level of communication with others on to a more enchanted plane, using the power of aroma …

Things to Do Every Day

☆ PRETEND EVERY DAY IS A BIRTHDAY. Each time you light a scented candle, concentrate for just a few seconds on the colour, and then a few more on the scent as it is released. Vividly imagine something you wish for: see it like a tiny movie actually happening, breathe in the colour and the smell, and say the words: *'This will be.'* And then, of course, when you blow out the candles, make the wish verbally again – just like you do with the candles on a birthday cake!

☆ A HAND-WRITTEN LETTER is very special in an age where most communications happen by e-mail or text. Next time you have an important note to write, for a 'thank you' or an invitation, make it scented. Choose a scent that is appropriate: look at the full list of oils at the end of this book for help *(see pages 89–93)*. If the card concerns a romantic invitation or note, the scent should be floral; if it concerns a party or business, go for a citrus smell; if it is to spread joy, you might choose a herbal scent. Choose a bottle of coloured ink, add six drops of the oil you like, shake the bottle and dip in that fountain pen. Add a few more scented petals to the envelope when you close. Imagine the magic you are making when it arrives: you are ensuring a positive and uplifting response, and it works miracles, believe me!

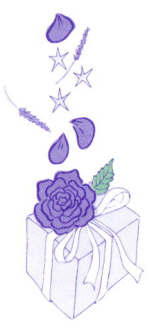

☆ When you WRAP A GIFT, do the same as above, and add a few scented flower buds to the parcel. Lavender and rose buds emerging from tissue paper along with a gift make the recipient feel so special, but also work an instant magic, subtly tightening the bond between you. And you can scent the wrapping paper first, placing a tissue infused with a few oils next to or inside the paper before you use it. Whenever you make up a package, always make a special wish for you and the recipient.

☆ The scent that comes in SHOWER AND BATH GELS is magic waiting to be released. Never miss the moment – every morning or evening – to visualize a magical goal coming true when you inhale the scent and take it into your open pores. When you have citrus aromas, which are frequently found even in supermarket gels, visualize a little extra monetary success. If the smells are rosy or other single note florals, visualize an emotional wish being granted: close your eyes tightly and smile as you think! If the scent is more herbal or cleansing (such as eucalyptus or rosemary), see yourself taking control of a difficult situation, being assertive. And if you have something you need to remember, use a basil-, geranium-, rosemary- or lavender-based cleanser, breathe it right in and go calmly over the facts you need to recall. Later, they will come flooding back to you as you smell your deliciously scented skin, and a tissue impregnated with one of these oils that you can sniff before a meeting or exam will help the information to flow smoothly.

☆ Have you got a CONFERENCE OR MEETING coming up where you will use typed material? If it is for business, use lemon, grapefruit or juniper oils in a blend you like, adding about eight drops neat to a cotton wool pad or ball; slip it inside the folder with the paper-work, and watch the brightness as you release the papers from their resting place. This works especially well if you have hand-outs or leaflets to distribute, as not only will they make an impression on your audience, but they will also lift the recipient's feelings of confidence in YOU! Pure magic! If the matter concerns something social – invitations and so on – use bergamot oil when men are included, and melissa (lemon balm) if it is all for women. You will receive such positive feedback …

☆ Need to have a really MAGICAL WORKING DAY? Perhaps you want to feel more alert or be noticed for your talents? Any lemon-scented oils (lemon oil, lemon balm, lemon pepper or lemon thyme) will increase your sunshine qualities and help you radiate gentle energy and goodness. Either put a few drops into warm water near a heater where you sit, or make up a room spray of fifteen drops lemon-scented oil in 100 ml (4 fl oz) spring water. Spritz every hour or so where you work; some firms have even found this increases keyboard efficiency and reduces errors! You'll soon get promoted.

☆ Want to make gentle LOVE-MAGIC every day? Whether you have a tired partner or just need a boost yourself after a stressful working shift, love can always use a helping hand from magical scents. For a romantic weekend at home or away with someone you want to leave hankering for you, shampoo and condition your hair the night before, following with a clear-water rinse of essential oils steeped in spring water. Try using scented geranium: it is romantic but also thought-provoking, and your beloved will look at you through changed eyes! Otherwise, orange-flower or rose are pretty hard to beat. This also leaves a fabulous scent on the pillow ...

☆ And more ROMANTIC SURPRISES? Spice up the air in your love nest: jasmine, neroli, rose, sandalwood and vanilla all speak the most seductive language on your behalf. Make a blend or use one note, and diffuse the oils into the area where you relax together. The same combination can be sprayed on to bedlinen to utter seductive invitations, and perfuming your tresses with any of these oils will make your intentions charmingly clear to your companion!

☆ And finally, for success and MAGICAL RESULTS AT SPORT or in a physically demanding task, make a blend of bergamot, cardamom, cedar- or sandalwood, juniper and any citrus oils. Put them in a dish in a warm area where you change: you will be full of courage, confidence and power before you step out into the arena. If you play a team game, make sure you spread the aroma widely enough for all to feel its benefits. This is very powerful magic indeed.

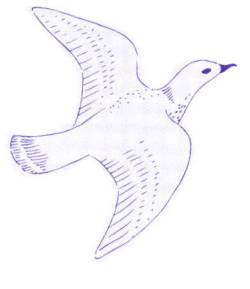

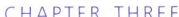
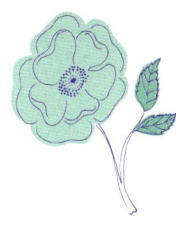

CHAPTER THREE

Love and Emotion

*As you are now beginning to think of scent as part of a magical
routine, we can explore different uses of aromatic oils, in spell rituals,
to embellish your emotional life. We all need help in this sphere sometimes: single
girls want to emit the right signals for a zingy new love affair, while those of us in
long-running partnerships can benefit from injecting a little amorous vigour into the
arena. We may need to deal with the crisis of getting over a love affair and find
a positive way to move forwards; or perhaps we are attracted to someone who will
always fall short of our hopes. In all these circumstances, magic ritual can erase
some of the problems, and aroma power will enhance the spell. In every case,
the scents introduced in this chapter will make us feel good about ourselves,
which is the start of all good relationships!*

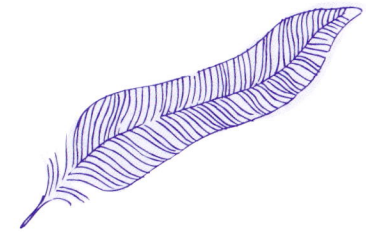

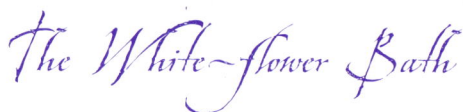

The White~flower Bath

Bathing is a common beginning in ritual to seeing and projecting a new self. This regime entices good feelings from yourself and beguiles your own spirit to soar and be loved.

Haven't met anyone who excites your appetite for love yet? Try this beautiful scented spell to help you signal to your inner self that you are ready, and to put out a message in a laid-back sort of way ...

YOU WILL NEED: *Petals from three fragrant roses (any colour)*
Paper towels
Tray
1 teaspoon sugar
Six to eight flowering heads of elderflower (or 1 tablespoon elderflower cordial if unavailable)
Large jar with a tight lid
1 pint full-cream milk
Wooden spoon
One white satin ribbon, about 50 cm (20 in) in length
Two white floating scented candles
Floating bowl for the candles
One fragrant white flower (whatever is in season, such as magnolia, gardenia, freesia, jasmine or rose)

WHAT YOU DO: Dry out your rose petals on paper towels, then place them on a tray and dust with sugar. Leave for one hour. Now place the elderflower heads (or elderflower cordial if you can't get the fresh flowers – but do try!) into the large jar. Pour the milk over the flowers (or cordial) and add the rose petals, with as much sugar as remains on the petals. Stir three times with a wooden spoon, saying: *'The rose and the elder grant to me, secrets of love, life and beauty.'* Gently shake the contents, and put them in a cool place. Let them steep for several hours (or overnight).

Run a bath, and pour the contents of the jar into the bath without straining them. The sugar will sweeten your skin and open it for the scent to enter the pores. Undress for your bath with some calm and ritual. Play some emotive music, and tie the ribbon around your brow. Now light the scented candles floating in a bowl beside your bath (take care where you place them!) and float the scented flower with the candle. Breathe in the scents, first from the flower, then from the bath, and imagine the white light and scent entering your whole self through the white ribbon round your forehead. Close your eyes and picture yourself tall, radiant and calm. Imagine you are capturing a new spirit of personal spark, and let your body drink in the physical and psychological treats. As you get out of the bath, see yourself as the goddess Venus – patron of beauty and love – arising from the sea.

This ritual is as appropriate to use just before taking yourself off to bed alone as it is before going out to see someone special, or attending a party where you hope to meet someone new. You are always worth the investment of time and psychological pampering. Performed regularly, this ritual will allow your physical beauty to emerge more and more strongly, and your confidence will shine! Love is in the air …

A Ritual to Counter Anxiety

This is a simple and effective way to battle the symptoms of anxiety in love,
and persuade the mind to feel more optimistic.

Love affairs sometimes go wrong for reasons of fear, or emitting 'stressed' vibes, even when you can attract a suitor easily. The reasons for this are usually a trained response to a series of let-downs in love, or perhaps in the original family unit. It is as though there is an accentuated response to the number of things that might go wrong. If this is a problem you recognize, this aromatic ritual offers a way to retrain your mind and help you exude more confidence and calm in a relationship.

YOU WILL NEED: *10 drops geranium oil*
10 drops lavender essential oil
10 drops bergamot oil
Diffuser (or 30 ml/1½ fl oz base oil, such as baby oil or sweet almond oil)
Photograph of yourself at a happy, relaxed moment
One fragrant flower
Tissues

WHAT YOU DO: Diffuse the oils in your burner, or blend them with a base oil and add them to a warm bath. Do this regularly, for at least seven days. For a few minutes each time, inhale the aroma and look at the photograph of yourself in a truly happy mood, when you felt good even if it were just for a frozen moment! Let the oils entice your mind to warm yellow-orange colours, like the sun; imagine that light around you in the picture, and then around you as you sit/stand physically now. Close your eyes, breathe in the scent and say: *'I can rise above doubts, and fly like a bird.'* You must repeat this simple mantra three times; do it every day, and keep the oils around you for at least a week (my grandmother would say that a whole moon cycle of twenty-eight days was best!). Finally, put a fragrant bloom of your choice next to your photograph, either in a vase or just across the picture.

Wear something sunshine-coloured for a month and sprinkle the oils onto a tissue to keep in your pocket. Whenever you are in contact with your love, or someone to whom you are attracted, sniff the tissue and smile. You'll soon get the hang of it.

And a variant:

If you sometimes ruin relationships by getting paranoid and angry yourself, or if you want to counter mutual anger in relationships, or even cope with unexpressed anger towards a loved one, do exactly as above, but substitute these oils: 5 drops rose otto oil, 5 drops camomile, 10 drops linden blossom. Use a photograph of yourself taken when you were serene and happy. Diffuse the oils for at least half an hour, breathe in the scent gently and imagine the serene you in the photo coming 'inside the soul' of the you in the here and now. Imagine green and pink colours surrounding you and protecting you. You should soon find the anger ebbing away, and a feeling of control and self-belief creeping back.

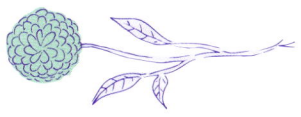

A Ritual to Remedy Emotional Loss

Ralph, a wise friend in Sydney who taught yoga and well-being classes, once expressed to me his view that emotional pain – that ache of the heart over a lost relationship – was possibly the worst pain there was. It is hard to disagree. This spell-ritual is not offering to bring someone back from the past; sometimes that is out of the question, particularly after bereavement. However, it will help to strengthen you against feelings of desolation and emptiness so that, over time, healing can occur and a new life can emerge.

YOU WILL NEED: *5 drops each of any four of the following oils: benzoin, hyacinth, neroli, rose maroc, rose otto, scented geranium, tuberose, vetiver*
Diffuser
White scented candle, especially rose-scented
An item that belonged to the person from whom you are parted
Shrub or small tree

WHAT YOU DO: For as many days or weeks as you need, burn any four of the oils above together in your diffuser. If you have actually lost someone through death, make sure to include vetiver or benzoin and one of the roses in the mix. Ensure that, as they diffuse, you spend time giving thought to the person from the past. Take half an hour if you can, smell the air, breathe gently and calmly, and see their face in your mind. Whatever the reason for your parting – either a broken relationship or another kind of loss – send them two beautiful thoughts concerning something special they did for, or with, you in your time together. Even if they were someone who has since hurt you, thank them for what was good: this is the only way to get over guilt or anger, and grow. Actually say the words 'thank you' while you think of them.

Also, each evening at a specific time (say between 8 and 9 o'clock, or similar), light the white fragrant candle in your private space. If possible, place the item from the person you have lost near the candle (taking care about its safety near the flame, of course). Say their name and think of them warmly for a moment, and then see yourself visually walking towards the light represented by the candle flame.

On a day that suits you, perhaps an anniversary, the first feasible weekend or even just the first free day of a new moon, sprinkle some of the oils into a hole in the ground (or a pot), where you can plant the tree or small shrub in honour of the best aspects of the person you loved and no longer have. The flowers on the plant should be pink if you lost a partner in a love relationship, mauve or blue if you have lost someone in the family, and white if your loss concerns a child in any way. Ask a friend to join you, if you like. The first step is to sprinkle the oils, and then place just one item from your lost love (a photograph would do fine if you have nothing else that you want to lose) in the hole before you plant the roots of the shrub or tree in the earth. Say out loud: *'May all that was beautiful, magical and special about our time continue to be part of us, and may you journey to a new sphere with peace.'*

Tend the plant well: it represents an idea and an actuality of what can never die, what will flourish in a different way, and a time that is closed for now. Whenever you need to, visit it and sprinkle some oils. The relationship will be changed, but with time a new grace will enter your spirit, and better fortunes will find you.

Spell to Cast Away Self-doubt

If you have begun a new relationship and want to make the feelings of excitement last, or if you don't even feel as though you can get off the blocks in love matters because your confidence is shaky or you are feeling shy, this spell will work wonders.

YOU WILL NEED: *Incense sticks (anything flower-based, such as jasmine, lavender, orange blossom, rose, and so on)*
A broom!
A deep-pink ribbon about 30 cm (12 in) long

WHAT YOU DO: Start on a full moon. Light your chosen incense in your home and, while it is burning, use your broom to do some actual sweeping. Tie the pink ribbon loosely around one wrist, and generate some real sweat with that besom. Begin at one end of the house and move through it, saying out loud as you sweep: *'I purify my house and my spirit. I sweep away sad and confused feelings. I clear a path for a new powerful me, rewarded in love. So mote it be!'* Sweep once through the house, then untie the ribbon and pass it once through the incense smoke. Over the wafting smoke, say these words once more.

Enact this calorie-burning ritual three times: once on a full moon, once on the three-quarter moon (i.e. a week later) and the third time one week later again. You are sweeping away negativity, hence the waning moon (which always rids us of unwanted emotions). After the new moon dawns around the time of the third sweeping, you had better get your wardrobe ready for some romantic excursions: a new life is arriving!

Lemon A-peel

If you have someone in your heart, but you're not sure if it's the real thing – or whether your feelings are reciprocated – this scented ritual might help. It is for anyone who wants to learn whether the one they love will satisfy their heart for some time, or let down their hopes. Don't worry if this seems a little odd in some ways! It is a very ancient ritual, and 'tried and true', as the saying goes. Lemon brings honesty …

YOU WILL NEED: *Lemon-scented shower gel or soap*
Lemon peel
Diffuser
Lemon and geranium essential oils

WHAT YOU DO: First thing in the day, wash yourself with a lemon-scented product. As you wash, breathe the aroma and picture your loved one's face. Gently towel dry. Next, take two small lemon peels and put them under your armpits for a few hours (yes, seriously: you may need to use plasters!). Keep them there as long through the day as you comfortably can (interesting early deodorant!).

At night, rub the end of your bed with the peels (don't argue: just do it!). Light your diffuser and scent the room with blended lemon and geranium oils. Read for half an hour while the scent diffuses. After lights out, picture your love's face as you close your eyes…. In your dreams, your love should come to you and offer you lemons or a gift, or present you with scented offerings. If you don't see him (or her), things look disappointing – unless they *actually* appear during the week with a fragrant gift! Fingers crossed.

A Fragrant Chemistry Lesson!

Be the perfect sex kitten at social soirees, girls!
(Sorry, boys: this is for the female witchlings only!)

Got a date after a twelve-hour working day? Find it impossible to be a sex goddess after a hard week in the office? Or maybe you simply want to bolster your passion and sex appeal for a party invitation? Well, we often make the most impact when we haven't tried too hard at all: there's something mysterious about a woman who's a little laissez-faire or enigmatic. If you perform the ritual below, you can go to all the fuss and trouble before you don your stilettos, and then exude just the right amount of ennui! Venus, goddess of love, rules the hour from 5 to 6 o'clock pm (an hour later in summer), so this is when you should start your ritual if possible.

YOU WILL NEED: *Glue*
One rose petal
Tuberose essential oil
1 teaspoon baby oil
10 drops either damiana or gingko essence (see pages 94–5 for stockists)
One glass champagne
Stockings
One white feather
2 drops unscented pheromone

WHAT YOU DO: Glue your rose petal to a calendar or date-diary on the date of a forthcoming special event, and say simply: *'Honour to Venus, Goddess of Love.'* Then, on the day itself, at the hour appointed above (or as near as possible), dilute three drops tuberose oil in the baby oil and then dab the blend on the inside and outside of each ankle and on each temple. Close your eyes and see yourself relaxed and in control.

Infuse ten drops damiana or gingko essence into a glass of champagne. Sip the drink, and use your own words to toast and honour Venus and the Moon. Lightly rub just behind each anklebone for a moment, and smell the fragrance deeply: this releases the sex kitten in you like nothing on earth. Recharge the champagne tonic throughout the evening (using ten drops of essence each time) and keep rubbing one foot against the other!

Put on some stockings (NOT tights!) and be careful with your perfumed hands if you are using thigh-highs: scent will encourage them to creep downwards. Remember to sip your champagne! Now spritz a little tuberose on to the feather, and put it in your purse (you can use it imaginatively later ...). Apply two drops of pheromone under your nose. It is unscented, but don't specially inhale it; it is the tuberose your nose should enjoy! Both scent and pheromone boost your own feel-good factor, enhancing your powers of attraction, and making you exude sensuality like a tigress.

Just before you go out, touch the rose petal on the calendar page, down the last few drops of champagne love-potion, and set forth! You are positively bursting with inner 'chi' (life energy), so let this do all the talking while you relax and feel quietly in control. The night ahead is all yours, even if your day began at dawn. Have fun, Cinderella!

Scented Love Wishes

These three spells are wonderful wishing rituals from our past. Wishes are intense thoughts, which work most often when an unbelievable strength of mind is focused upon them. The powerful use of aromatic oils puts our brain in gear to generate high-voltage positive thoughts that can become amazing actualities. The simple rituals revolve around a little herb or fruit with an intense flavour and/or scent. These crystallize the magical strength of our wishes, and set them off in turn, mysteriously, into the ether ...

My grandmother had a treasure trove of these delightful rituals and always warned me to be ever so careful what I wished for – for it would certainly come true. Later she suggested that my wishes might not remain the same as those of my younger self, so I was to pick carefully. Here is a trilogy from her personal collection of best-loved, tried-and-true scented wish-rituals, all concerning love matters. And do they work? Get that diffuser ready to see ...

Lavender love wish for a headache sufferer

When you have a headache that simply won't shift, your love (or an admirer) is trying to tell you something! Try this ritual with dried lavender sprigs ...

WHAT YOU DO: Use lavender oil on its own, or blended with rose geranium, and add up to ten drops to warm water in your diffuser. Make a mild infusion of lavender tea, using 1 tablespoon dried lavender in 600 ml (1 pint) boiling water, and sweeten with ½ teaspoon honey. Brew for ten minutes, enjoying the lavender in the air as it steeps; then sip the tea slowly. While you are drinking, ask who is thinking of you and what they wish to say to you. Look into the cup, and you should soon see the face of your love or some new admirer who is thinking of you. While you drink your tea and inhale the diffused oil, the message will come through and your headache will disappear.

Rose love wish for a singleton

This ancient ritual has accompanied deep feelings of love from countless young lasses. Why not try it yourself … and I think countless young lads might try it too?

WHAT YOU DO: On Midsummer Night (21 June), heat some rose maroc or rose otto perfume oil in warm water in your diffuser; breathe in the scent deeply, close your eyes and go into your garden or wherever you can grow your own flowers (you may need to get a pot-grown rose bush for a balcony or window). Now you must gather a rose, but without speaking a word to anyone. Clasp it to your heart, minding the thorns, and make a wish for happiness in love. Walk backwards, if possible, back into your bedchamber (doesn't that sound romantic? But don't trip over!). Fold the rose up in a sheet of clean white paper, making sure that you can still smell the diffusing scent of the rose. Set it aside carefully until midwinter (21 December) or Christmas Day. On that day, light the rose oil in the burner again and wear the dried rose pinned to a jacket or coat, or even placed in a locket. On this day you will have a special declaration of love.

Apple love wish for divination

This is an old device for telling whether your love is true. If you can't find apple-wood or apple fragrance oil, use another wood oil like rosewood or sandalwood, and add some apple peel to the warm water in the diffuser.

WHAT YOU DO: On Hallowe'en, or at Yule or New Year, scent the air strongly with apples – either with a diffuser into which you place some geranium and apple oils, or with an apple-scented candle. Next, take some apple pips and throw them one by one into an open fire or barbecue. Address someone you love with each pip, envisaging their face and saying to yourself: *'If you love me true, pop and fly; if not, lie quiet and die.'* If the pip bursts in the heat, or makes a noise, it is a certain proof of love …

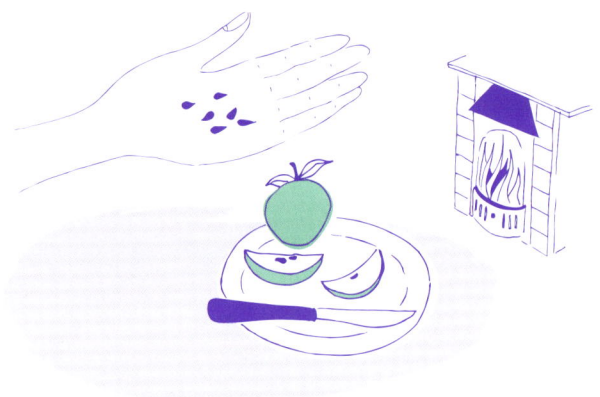

A Brew to Encourage a Tongue~tied Admirer

A flower exudes its blissful fragrance unashamedly – to be ravished!
It cries to its pollinator to kiss it awake with procreative life. And, by borrowing
the scent and the very heart of the flower's spirit in this spell, so do we!

This is just the spell to perform if you have had your eye on someone who is – as yet – too shy or hesitant to make a move in your direction. If you correctly think there might be some degree of interest on their side, this will do the trick and get things moving!

YOU WILL NEED: *A bottle of coloured ink – red or pink hues for preference*
2 drops scented geranium oil, blended with 2 drops lavender oil
A small dish (to use as an inkwell, to save scenting the whole bottle of ink)
A fountain pen
A piece of coloured spell paper – no more than 5 x 1 cm (2 x ½ in) wide
Three roses, coloured as you please
Seasonal greenery, including any fresh herbs such as lemon balm,
rosemary or oregano
A small piece of florists' wire
A scented candle

WHAT YOU DO: Scent a small amount of the ink by blending it with the drops of essential oils in a small dish. Fill the pen with it, and write the name of the person you like so much on the piece of spell paper. While the name is drying thoroughly on the paper, start to make a tiny fragrant wreath from the roses and greenery, using the wire as a base. Weave the flowers into and around it at roughly equal intervals, until they are secure. Before you have finished the circlet, you should hide the name in amongst the herbs. All the while you are weaving away, you should sing or hum a love song that you like – but it should be light and flirty and not too binding in its message!

When the pretty object is complete, say your friend's name aloud, and honour their spirit and the qualities you like, along with their right to choose to take up your invitation to know you better, *freely*. Do not coerce with your words, but simply invite, flirtatiously. Finish by placing the circlet around the base of the candle (but make sure the candle cannot catch light with the herbage, by putting it safely on a heatproof dish and allowing enough room for the flowers to stand well away from the flame). Now light the candle; as you do, say your name and your friend's name, and ask that a light be kindled between you to see if there is a spark that can grow. Breathe in the scent as it is released from the ink, the flowers and the candle.

Allow the candle to burn for just five minutes, and then extinguish it. Take the circlet and put it somewhere safe – by the bed or in your living area. Ask it to look beautiful for a few days and emit powerful magic on your behalf. Before the week is up, you should discover whether there is any potential between you!

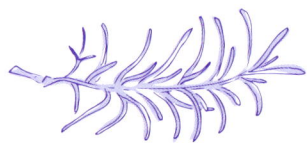

A Concoction to Calm Mood Swings

Sometimes we behave very irrationally. It is a task and a half for the most patient of partners to cope when we have complete mood blowouts! So, here is a blissful scented spell to calm you down when you are about to let fly. If the mood is caused at base level by pressures from the outside world, drinking this hedonistic brew before bedtime will help you dream of and understand more about the causes, and how they can be dealt with. After performing this, you will awaken to a new inner beauty in the eyes of your loved one, and freshly excite their feelings for you …

YOU WILL NEED: *Ingredients for tea: 1 tablespoon fresh rose petals or dried apothecary's rose; 1 teaspoon jasmine or jasmine tea (but fresh flower is best); 1 vanilla pod; 1 cinnamon stick; 1 teaspoon fresh or dried vervain*
A pretty pink (or chintzy) china teacup
One rose-scented candle
1 drop benzoin oil in 5 ml carrier oil
A rose-pink satin ribbon, about 1 m (3⅓ ft) in length

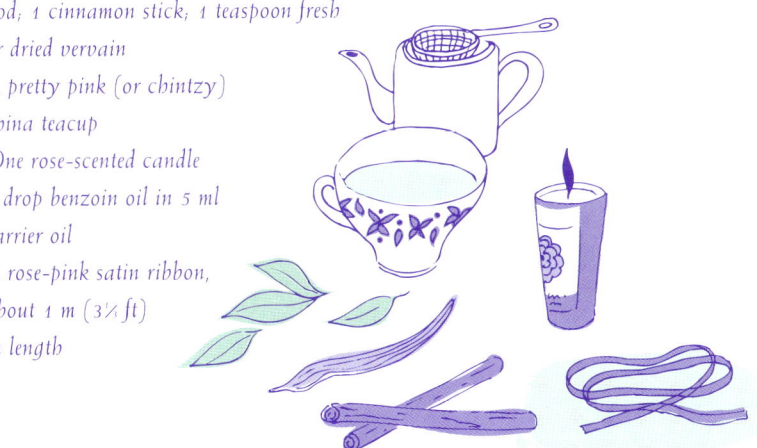

WHAT YOU DO: As the moody barometer rises, make a brew of this delicious concoction before retiring to bed (whether or not you are alone …). Brew the tea ingredients together in boiling water for ten minutes, then strain into your teacup. Before you sip, light the candle, massage your temples very gently with the diluted benzoin oil and tie the ribbon loosely around your waist. (Share this with your bemused partner if you have company!) Sip, and think of beautiful, romantic things. See yourself calm, happy, serene and riding on the crest of a wave of emotional contentment. The more strongly you can visualize, the more effective the spell will be.

The tea will incite you to amazing, inspired, even quite psychic dreams, and you will wake with a look of romantic wildness and fresh beauty. You will also find your sulkiness dissipates, leaving a glowing serenity in its place. And a renewed and revitalized love affair, in all likeliness!

Magic to Keep a New Relationship Blooming

When you fall in love, your feet don't touch the ground. But it is difficult to perpetuate that feeling, and keep the romance of an affair kindled as familiarity grows. From the first day of your 'new' and beautiful love life, if possible – and at least once a week after that – try this wake-up regime to create a day of beautiful romance that unfolds around you and embraces your growing bond together.

A sexy, scented shower

YOU WILL NEED: Group 1: *1 teaspoon ground almonds; 1 teaspoon lemon juice (for oilier skins) OR 1 tablespoon avocado (for normal and drier skins); 1 tablespoon natural yoghurt; 3 leaves fresh basil, chopped*
Small dish
Group 2: *juice of half a cucumber; 2 drops basil oil; 2 drops scented geranium oil; 2 caplets of starflower oil (borage); 1 tablespoon baby shampoo*
Lidded bottle
A few scented flowers (from garden or market)
Yellow or green bottles or vases

WHAT YOU DO: Blend the first group of ingredients in a small dish with your middle finger; this will become a face-mask. Blend the second group in a lidded bottle as a shampoo. Apply the face-mask in the morning, just for five minutes while you shower with the shampoo. Make these fresh each time, as it only takes a few minutes. Arrange the flowers in the bottles or vases around the bathroom. Make sure you breathe in the colour from the flowers and glass, for yellow and green kick you off with great vitality. The basil sparks the brain and also fires the juices for love, so that you exude the right elements for attractiveness in the broadest sense, both from within and without.

A light breakfast for love and beauty

Every woman needs lemon balm for her sensuality – and any man who takes it will understand his lady a little better! Yoghurt and mint both sweeten the breath and make the skin glow, while the lemon balm feeds your womanliness, so you exude very subtle but tangible sexuality. After your scented shower, share this breakfast with your love (or alone is fine, too!).

YOU WILL NEED: *150 ml (6 fl oz) natural low fat yoghurt*
100 ml (4 fl oz) fresh orange juice
One sprig mint
Two sprigs fresh lemon balm (grow a pot of lemon balm just for this recipe)
Ice

WHAT YOU DO: Blend all the ingredients together in a processor and enjoy. Make time for this breakfast even if you have nothing else with it (though, of course, on a weekend it is bound to invite subsequent courses to follow …). This is a light breakfast, but it gets your metabolism moving, which is essential for health, beauty and continuing romance. Cheers!

Scented Omen to Mend a Disagreement

Try this on weekends, Friday evenings, in summer, or to 'make up' after a fight.

This is something to do as often as you can make time, with whatever fresh flowers are in season. Choose essential oils to match some of the flowers you use. But always use it if one of you has been quarrelsome, and vary the mixture.

YOU WILL NEED: *A fresh-picked posy of sensual herbs and flowers mixed: try blending freesias, lavender, love-in-a-mist, marjoram, peonies, roses, scented geranium leaves, sweet peas, violets – anything you can get your hands on that is scented*
A blend of aromatic oils in carrier oil: choose any that match at least one 'note' from the fresh flowers and herbs
Small scented votive candle (try rose or green tea)

WHAT YOU DO: Tie an informal aromatic bunch of these blooms and leave it on freshly washed bedlinen, near to the pillows, as a surprise for your partner. Meanwhile, make up a massage potion with twenty drops of your chosen oils in a carrier oil of almond or primrose. Remember that at least one of the oils should match a flower or herb. And just before you retire to bed together, light a votive candle. All of these scents relieve guilt, trigger joy and pleasure, and help us release our natural endorphins to make us feel good about ourselves.

I think you know the rest …

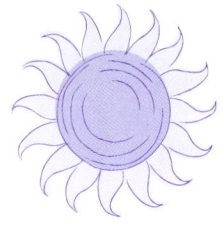
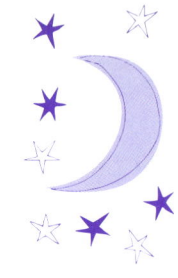

CHAPTER FOUR

Taking Charge

*Marrying aromatic oils with magical ritual can help us to take charge
of problem areas in our lives. Magical ritual has always been principally
concerned with gentle and oft-repeated mantras that induce a self-hypnotic state;
chanting, symbolic ritual and the release of natural spirits in plants and herbs have
been central to this ritual. Scent, as we now understand, 'clinches' the effect, leaving
a powerful and re-energized mental state from which we can write new chapters
in our life story. So here we will learn how to tackle loner tendencies that
prevent us from full social ease and interaction; to be more assertive
and cope with tests in life; to be more confident, creative and happy.
In every case, the aromatic elements will fortify our will
and offer pleasures of their own.*

Spell for a Loner or Those Who Love a Loner

The hardest wall to break through can be with those we love who don't want to give up single-life habits, or who are shy of exposing their feelings to others and are thus unused to communicating closely with anyone. It can ruin relationships, whether love, business, friendship, or even with our family members. Anyone can become set in their ways. Or, perhaps it's you who worries about adjusting to being in a couple after some time alone, or finds giving up your delicious self-sufficiency for other people – however enticing – a bridge too far? Shyness can be crippling, and paranoia even more so. Loneliness can seem an unconquerable barrier to happiness. Try this ritual to entice either yourself, or a loner you care for, out of the habit of being alone.

YOU WILL NEED: *A photograph frame that holds two pictures: one of you – or the person you care for – on your/their own, and the other of you and your love together (it doesn't matter if the photo is of you both as part of a bigger group, if that's all you have)*
Two unscented candles, in a blue colour hue
Any three of the following oils: benzoin, bergamot, camomile, helichrysum, melissa, narcissus, neroli

WHAT YOU DO: On a new moon, place the photo frame on a small table or window-sill, which serves as an altar. Next, scent and light the candles: using one or more of the oils from the list, light both the candles and let them burn for about five minutes until the wax around the wick is molten. Blow out the flames. Add a few drops of your chosen oil/s to the wax while it is liquid. Wait another five minutes for it to harden. Then place the candles near the picture frame, and relight them.

Once the scent starts to be released, say a benediction addressing both your-self and your loved one. If it is *you* who is the loner, say the following: '[your loved one's first name] – *I honour you when we are together, and enjoy our shared time. Long may it reign. I also ask, though, that you respect my own will and my personal time, as I will try to respect the time you may need when you want quiet time or need to retreat from others. Singly and together, let us prosper. Blessings on us.'*

If your love or friend is the loner, say this: '[their first name] – *I honour you and comprehend your need for privacy and solitude. You may be shy and protective of your own time and space sometimes. I also honour you when you give of yourself to make good company with me and other friends. Don't be afraid of sharing either laughter or silence. I will respect you as your needs dictate, as I ask you do for me. Singly and together, let us grow closer and more at ease. Blessing be to us both.'*

Keep the candles with the framed photographs. Light the flames whenever you are together, taking care to recharge the scents as necessary. Use these same oils in a diffuser, as unobtrusively as possible, to lift the atmosphere in your most relaxing room and make a gentle and supportive environment in which affection for others and social confidence can grow. Regular use of these scents, and the occasional repetition of the ritual, will assist any relationship or friendship to blossom, with greater aware-ness of the individual needs of yourself and others. They will also ease the feeling of isolation whenever you (or your friend) are alone.

Quick Creativity Spell

Got to deliver a piece of original work? Can't think of anything to do or say?
Follow this recipe for a bright spark of imagination!

YOU WILL NEED: *Vase of fresh flowers, all lemon and orange colours (freesias, poppies,*
roses, sunflowers, tulips, and so on)
Baby bath oil or foam
10 drops each geranium, neroli, and
either bay, carnation, juniper, mimosa
or sandalwood essential oils

WHAT YOU DO: Set the flowers where you
can enjoy them from your bath. Blend the
bath oil/foam with your choice of oils and
add it to the bath as it fills. Before you get
into the bath, touch your belly button firmly
and circle it three times clockwise. Then
jump into the tub and imagine the colour
from the flowers penetrating right into the
centre of your mind, sending shards of the
same coloured light around your brain. Relax.
Take your time. When you emerge, thoughts
will suddenly jump and fly!

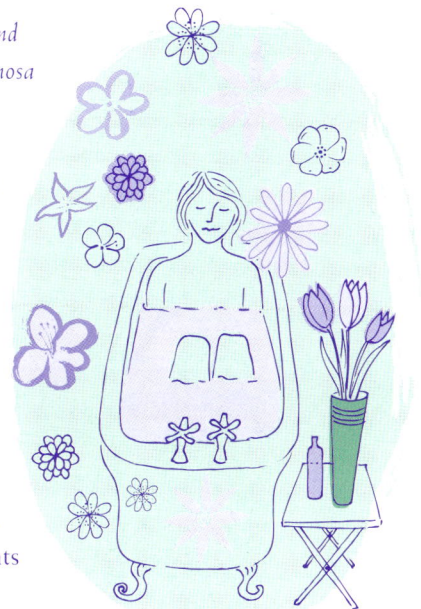

A Ritual for Assertiveness

Assertiveness means being able to say what you want to say, in a collected fashion, to others. It might be about business, money, rights, love, or just standing up for your own opinion. It might almost be a matter of integrity. Certainly, if you can be productively assertive – rather than just grouchy or merely aggressive – you are more likely to get what you need and find life and tough situations more manageable. Use the aroma power of the oils as often as you like, and repeat this ritual at least once each month until you begin to notice that you are not the passive person you might once have been!

YOU WILL NEED:
Calming music
5 drops each of three of the following oils: bergamot, cedarwood, coriander, cubeb (mae chang), cypress, lime, ormenis flower
Diffuser
A red silk handkerchief or scarf
A photograph of someone who most makes you shrink from speaking your mind (it might be a parent, an ex-lover, or a current one, or even a stern boss who treats you like a child)

WHAT YOU DO: You need to confront the demon of your past – whomever made you feel small and weak. Put on some gentle music that speaks straight to your soul (this might be anything from Gregorian Chant to Enrique Iglesias, although heavy rock might not be the best choice – choose something melodic and inspiring!). Next, diffuse your chosen oils (fifteen drops in total) in warm water in the burner. While holding on to the red silk fabric, take up the photo of the 'bully' in your past and address them eloquently and simply, looking straight into their eyes as you speak: *'Do you know how you curbed my spirit and my soul? Prevented my words from taking flight? For whatever reason you behaved this way, that reason and weakness was YOUR problem, and is no longer mine. I reject your value judgement, I let you go, and I let it be.'* Stroke the silk, breathe in the colour and the scents, and forgive the person who hurt you.

Do this about three times over two or three months, but diffuse the oils and stroke the red silk as often as you need to face anyone who has 'power' over you. After a few months you will find that you are quite strong and brave. Get out there and say what you need to!

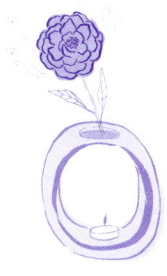

Spell for Exams or Tests

Continuing on from your greater self-assertion, this is the way to confront any day when you have an examination or a major trial to get through.

The spell helps you to recall facts easily, keeps you calm and in control of your information, and gives you clarity. Worth trying for even young children, it will be invaluable to teenagers taking regular tests, or anyone who needs to be convincing with words or information.

YOU WILL NEED: *Note cards or filing cards*
Lavender and geranium essential oils
Lavender or geranium scented candle
A picture postcard of a scene or place you like
A soft powder puff or velvety fabric square

WHAT YOU DO: Assemble all the information you have to cover in your meeting, test or exam. Revise your facts properly: for this, there is no substitute! Then, to make the details sink in, reduce your larger points to a few very simple sentences on a series of filing cards. Dab a drop of lavender oil in one corner of each card and geranium on the other. As many nights as possible before the bid or test, light the scented candle and sit for half an hour; look at the postcard, and then breathe in the scent while going over the points on each filing card, one at a time. Read each one, then say it out loud, and then tell it to the candle while inhaling its scent and that of the oils on the card. When you have done this calmly for about thirty minutes, stroke both your temples with a powder puff or velvet cloth. Rest. Repeat each night that you can before the test comes. On the day itself, put the oils on a tissue, the puff in your pocket, and the postcard somewhere you can glance at it just before you start (this will help to relax your mind). As soon as you breathe the tissue, you'll be off: whatever information you have absorbed will come flooding back. Use this ritual often and your memory will improve too.

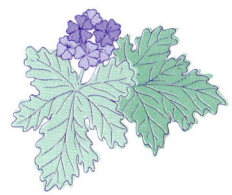

Conjuring Confidence

And, in a similar way to the previous spell, confidence can be sparked by feeling more 'knowing'. The by-products of confidence are manifold: you are more attractive to others, more successful and more fun to be with. Try this …

YOU WILL NEED: *One white candle*
A mirror
Lime, orange or coriander incense sticks and holder

WHAT YOU DO: Light the candle and sit in front of the mirror. Light the incense and wave it once across the glass, then burn it in a holder very close to you, where you can see your own reflection and the smoke. Take three shorter breaths and one longer one, while inhaling the scent. Say: *'I am architect of my own future. I will be blessed.'* See yourself glowing and successful, and look at the flame of the candle. Repeat seven times over a week. Whenever you need an extra pinch of confidence, burn the incense and then set forth!

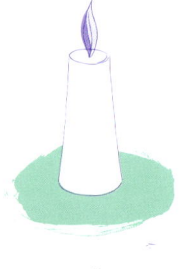

Potion for Joy and Happiness

A nice-and-naughty love and happiness potion, to keep the temperature up when you're feeling cold, bored, sad or have a flat battery!

This potion works quite fast and may rescue you from a sense of sadness or oppression. Do it as often as you can, to generate joyous emotions for yourself.

YOU WILL NEED: *2 drops each clove, jasmine and orange oils*
Diffuser
Sugar cube
3 drops gingko essence or tincture (see pages 94–5 for stockists)
Martini glass or champagne flute
An orange
Champagne or sparkling wine

WHAT YOU DO: Heat the oils in warm water in your diffuser. Allow the sugar to absorb the ginkgo essence, then drop it into the glass. Squeeze over half the orange, then top the glass with champagne. Decorate the rim with an orange slice, and serve very well chilled. Sniff the air, drink the brew and things will soon look wonderful to you (and to anyone with you)! If you do this in the evening, for instance, affairs could shortly warm up between you and your love. Otherwise, just enjoy it as a cocktail when you need a pick-me-up (far better than a G&T!).

Peace and Positivity: A Meditation

To enjoy peace and tranquillity truly, we would need to influence all the powerful men and women who make decisions for us in the world at large. This isn't really easy to achieve! However, we *can* place ourselves in a bubble of retreat, and experience our own private grace and peace. Crises happen to everyone; it's how you handle them that's important. Try this meditation exercise to draw a veil of calm over you.

YOU WILL NEED: *Rock rose (or wild rose) flower essence*
100 ml (4 fl oz) spring water
25 drops in total of frankincense, geranium, melissa, spikenard and yarrow
oils, blended to your taste
A spray bottle (such as those used for misting plants, or perhaps a perfume
atomizer)
A pale pink satin ribbon

WHAT YOU DO: You need to experiment here, because feelings of peace are individually induced. Take time to find a moment when you can be quiet and uninterrupted – play gentle music if you like – and take a few drops of your chosen rose essence according to the manufacturer's instructions. Now make up a facial spray by mixing the spring water with your blend of oils. Shake them up in your spray bottle and mist your face very gently. Take up your pink satin ribbon and look deeply at its colour before tying it around your forehead. Close your eyes, breathe in the scent and imagine a ball of pale pink to mauve light spiralling inside your tummy, very gently.

Gradually, imagine the light rising all the way up your body to your forehead, spreading the colour through every nerve. Catch the scent again, and relax. Do this for about five to ten minutes and then spray your face once more before you finish.

Do this again just before bedtime and it will lull you into an overwhelmingly peaceful sleep. When you are having trouble sleeping, use the oils as a spray on either your face or pillow, and then tie the ribbon around your wrist. Starting at your feet, imagine the pale pink colour, like a light, gradually touching every nerve and relaxing every muscle, from your feet to your knees to your thighs, and slowly on up your whole body. When you reach your head, say quietly and drowsily to yourself: *'Now I may rest, and wake only when and as I need to. Good night,* [and call yourself by your own name].' This acts as a meditative self-hypnosis to ease your mind into peaceful sleep. (Shh … good night!)

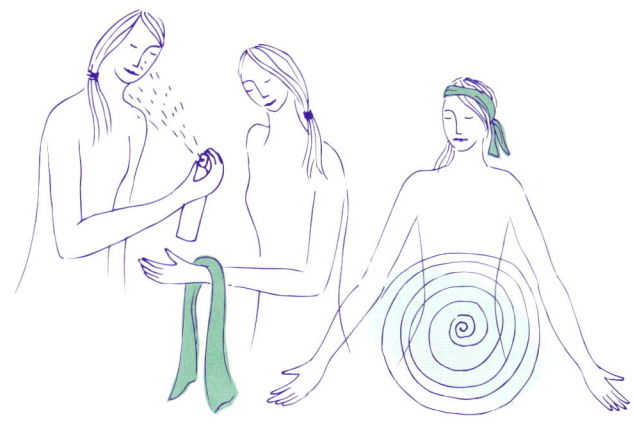

Scented Self-esteem

*Whatever size, shape, colour, earner or intellect you are, this ritual is a good way to
shake your own hand and enjoy meeting your real self!*

Our self-worth and self-image are crucial to our path through the world. We are tested,
contradicted and redefined by others who see us as they wish to, and it is sometimes
difficult to hang on to the best part of ourselves as *we* see it. Nor do we need to fit in
with any single cultural 'norm': our uniqueness is a divine gift, surely?

YOU WILL NEED: *Your favourite underwear (do you wonder what's coming?)*
*20 drops of any one of the following oils: gardenia, hyacinth, mandarin,
myrtle, rose maroc, vetiver*
Rose petals or lavender buds

WHAT YOU DO: Wait for a waxing moon, any time from new moon to the day
before full. Choose a relaxed day, when you have nothing to hurry for and no one
waiting on or watching you. Now, wash your favourite underwear – whatever is the
nicest colour, or has the nicest feel, in your whole lingerie drawer. (If nothing quite
matches this description, treat yourself to something new NOW!) Treat it as the most
special of delicate articles in a handwash; don't just fling it in the machine as though
it were ten years old and past its prime! After the soap is virtually washed out, scent
some warm water by adding twenty drops of your favourite oil from the list. Use this
oil blend as the final rinse, leaving the items to soak up the fragrance for about ten

minutes. Squeeze out gently and dry carefully – don't rush through a tumble dryer!

Have a shower while you wait. When your underwear is dry and still warm, get dressed into it (and a bathrobe if you like) and breathe in the aromatic sensuality from the lingerie. Vividly imagine both the scent and its flower or fruit entering right into your soul, and say: *'I am the one and only, special and unique, not perfect but precious, ME!'* Now sit on your bed and throw a few rose petals or lavender buds over yourself, as though you had just got married. Repeat the words: *'I am the one and only …'.* You should see yourself drenched in sunshine and light, scented, soulful, sassy and self-valuing.

Perform this simple ritual as often as possible: once a month is not too often and once a year not nearly enough. Your best underwear should be for you and not only for one special observer. And the delicious scent, once you have selected it, should become your signature aroma for self-esteem. If you want to use it often, and in many circumstances, try finding a commercial perfume based on the same single note for everyday wear. But always keep this one special oil for a ritual of self-anointing, as it were, for your magical self-image to soar.

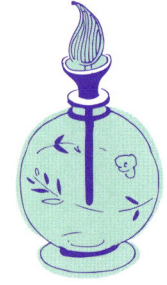

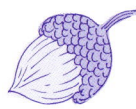

CHAPTER FIVE

Prosperity

Who said, 'Money has no smell'? I have heard that it was the Emperor
Nero, or possibly Trajan, who put a tax on public lavatories by charging
the proverbial penny. But I think that prosperity has a definite aroma. We can
smell success, and affluence may be fragrant. Equally, anyone or anything that
prospers is fragrant – usually from a designer bottle. In magic ritual, there are scents
that have always been associated with material prosperity, particularly yarrow,
hyssop and peony, but there are others too, each with a subtle spirit to attract reward
and encourage happiness in your professional life. We will examine them in this
chapter, and look at how you can use the power of aromatic oils to feel lucky, thrive
in your business or career, feel job-fulfilled and attract good fortune. It is not a
chapter addressing greed, for that is too much imbalance, but it will certainly
invite Providence to watch over you – and subsequently create more
pleasure in all work-related matters.

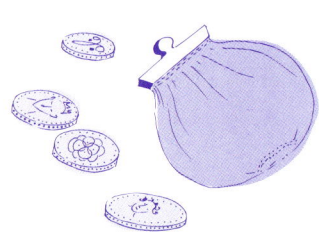

A Ritual to Attract Success

Never leave home for an important appointment concerning career or finance without an acorn in your pocket! If you don't live near an obliging oak, ask a jeweller to make a silver acorn for you. Always keep it near you to encourage material success, even to the extent of putting it on a keyring or attaching it to the zip of your purse. And then there's the scent ...

YOU WILL NEED: *Oak-moss essential oil*
Oak leaves – a handful, or even just one if you can't find many
A new coin purse
A coin
An acorn for your pocket or your key chain

WHAT YOU DO: This is the important part, as it is all in your mind. On a new moon – brand new if possible – run a bath and sprinkle in several drops of the oak-moss oil, together with the leaves. Soak in the tub for a while; as you do, imagine your work life and career aims keeping you very busy indeed. Hear the phone ring in your mind, with a voice saying you've been promoted, offered a job you want or been given a pay rise. If you own your own business, imagine it is thriving and that you are receiving phone calls constantly.

Inhale deeply, breathing in the scent of the oak moss. With each breath, see a few coins clinking into your purse and your pocket. As you emerge from the bath, say: *'A new life, of prosperity from rewarding work I enjoy, is dawning.'*

After your bath put two drops of oak-moss oil neat into your coin purse. Take any silver-coloured coin into moonlight and 'charge it up' from the light. Ask the lovely lady of the moon (Diana, or Epona to the Celts) – ancient provider who governs the hunt and thus procures sustenance – to favour you. Ask that your purse always have enough, and a little over. And then put your acorn into your new purse, once more inhaling the aromatic properties of the lucky oak-moss oil as you do so.

From now on, see yourself as lucky. Expect little bonuses and enough work to keep you busy in a position you enjoy. And you will go forth and prosper …!

A bonus charm

Whenever you have a very important meeting or interview, dilute 5 drops oak-moss oil in 25 ml (1 fl oz) spring water and spray on to an oak leaf to pin on your jacket. If you can't find an oak leaf, use a camellia or willow leaf instead.

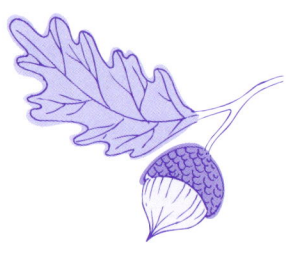

Flowers of Success

This is a sweet and special benediction to offer someone who has opened a business or started a new job. That person, of course, can be you!

YOU WILL NEED: *A few drops geranium oil and yarrow or hyssop oil*
One wide golden-yellow ribbon
Paper and pen
A shiny new pin
Bunch of flowers comprising: blue cornflowers, carnations (lemon-through-white colours), irises, peonies, sweet peas and white roses
Plenty of greenery (especially eucalyptus or mimosa, which is available for much of the year and is highly fragrant)

WHAT YOU DO: Dab the aromatic oils on to the ribbon. Write a note to wish 'blessings and blissful bounty' on the new job, etc., and pin it to the ribbon. Gather together the flowers and greenery in a bunch, then secure the ribbon around the flowers.

Give the flowers to the recipient with a smile (if it's you, smile as you put the stems in water, keeping them tied). Keep them there for a week (until they fade), and then preserve the flowers as a pot pourri. Take off the blooms and discard only the browned petals. Add salt and orris powder to make a pot pourri; air the petals and add a few drops of the oils as they dry out. Keep it in an open container where you work, with the silver pin hidden in the petals. Stir with one finger once a week, and ask for prosperity. Refresh the oils often (and add fresh petals!), and luck will smile on you!

A Ritual to Overcome Passivity

Francis Bacon once said: 'A wise man will make more opportunities than he finds.' It is easy to get into a groove with work, become apathetic and then almost frightened to change things. Before you know it, you no longer have the heart for your work, but feel unable to start in a new direction. Or it may be that a passive disposition is disabling you from feeling ambitious, getting promoted or saying that you would like to try a role that is more challenging. This ritual will help to boost your dynamism for work, and get you to where you really, really want to be!

YOU WILL NEED: *An oregano plant*
A coloured plant pot
A ribbon to tone with the pot
Incense – or oils to diffuse – from the following list: bay, jasmine, patchouli or ylang ylang

WHAT YOU DO: For this you need a growing plant in your work environment. Growing plants actually infuse life into their spaces: they are essential for any place where the energy currently feels a bit flat. So choose a small oregano plant and a decent-sized pretty pot to grow it in. The greens of the plant and its excellent aroma, which aids concentration and a feeling of overall vitality, are part of the blessing. However, the colour of the pot also has an important role to play. The idea is to lift your energy beyond the passive state, so you need to start by thinking of red, and then moving towards either purple or yellow. This means you can choose a pot that is of really warm pinks (quite high voltage, like cerise) or sunshine hues (red through orange). All of these will actually lift your pulse rate when you look at them for a few moments. If you can't find a pot this colour, create one: paint a terracotta pot in a colour from this range that fits in with your workspace decor.

Now you must 'charge' the atmosphere with your chosen scent. At least once a week, burn a stick of incense (with *sensitivity* for anyone near your work area, of course!) or diffuse a little oil. You may find that your colleagues are delighted to share the olfactory pleasures, and you can tell anyone who asks that studies prove the use of essential oils at work increases efficiency and concentration. So there!

Every day that you need to be especially energetic at work, tie the ribbon around the pot and say: *'I rise to the challenges ahead, and I make a neat, controllable parcel of my worries. I will emerge gently victorious.'* This is something you can do whenever you are under extra pressure; gradually you will find that you become more proactive in your work life, more rewarded for that, and happier with everything you do – in other words, prosperous! Look after that oregano plant – and long may it thrive!

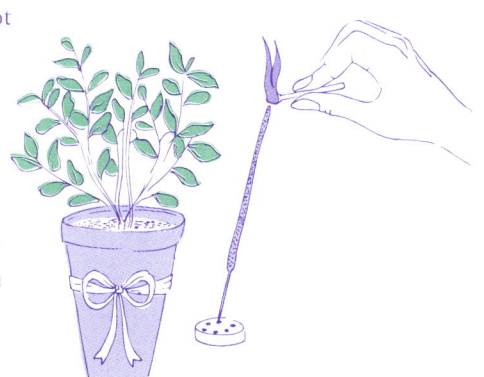

Spell to Increase Energy and Financial Luck

Dynamism at work and luck with money go hand in hand. This spell boosts your energy to deal with overwork, even near the point of burnout, and at the same time creates an aura of luck around you. Just see how well it works ...

YOU WILL NEED: *A small plant pot or tub*
Two or three plants of growing herbs: basil, bay, lemon balm, lemon verbena, marjoram, oregano, rosemary, scented geranium
Nutmeg essential oil
A whole nutmeg for your pocket or bag

WHAT YOU DO: Plant up the pot with your chosen herbs – opt for those you can get easily, and whose aromatic properties you like. As you plant, say: *'My luck will grow, my powers will flow.'* See yourself happy in your job.

AT WORK: take the tub anywhere you can leave it safely – in a tea-break space, for instance – and touch one different leaf on every break. Breathe in the aroma and see yourself literally flying through your day (go on – imagine yourself on a broom if you like!).

AT HOME: diffuse some nutmeg essential oil one day in every week – perhaps Sunday or Monday night. When you are worrying about money, rub the whole nutmeg in your pocket or bag and use a little more nutmeg in your food. Watch what happens.

Scented Wishes for Prosperity and Good Fortune

Just like the earlier set of wishing spells in Chapter Three, this trio of wish rituals are a legacy from my granny, who was a nineteenth-century wise-woman of the old school. She believed that anything we really wished for – with concentrated thought and ritual – would manifest. So, as she advised, choose your wishes very carefully in case you find out later that they were not what you wanted after all! The following three wishes are for luck with money and work.

Mint wish concerning money

Mint will bring you increased confidence, clarity and luck with both work and money.

WHAT YOU DO: Wear a sprig of mint pinned to a lapel, or tucked into your bodice or bra. It will not only bring you luck and confidence, but also protect you from the attentions or bad temper of anyone you don't like in the work arena: perhaps an ogre of a manager or an amorous pest who won't stop eyeing you inappropriately. If you are worried you may be set upon by an unwanted suitor, or bothered by a grumpy boss or colleague, dab a drop of peppermint oil in your hair, as well as placing a sprig of mint in your underwear. Play with your hair as you talk to them, and they will understand by magic that they need to respect your integrity and strength.

Also, wearing a mint leaf when you enter a competition or prize draw can help you attract luck. And if you have an indecent pile of bills to find the means to pay, take one coin of value, tape a piece of mint to it, and say: *'I wish to mint more money just to help with these bills. So mote it be.'* Then breathe in the scent from the leaf. During the following week, diffuse a little mint oil through your home for around an hour or so each night. Somehow, more money will find a way into your pocket to ease your worries. You'll see …

Scented strawberry wish

If you want to have an especially lucky day – and it might not just be luck in terms of money or business – go to bed the night before with this simple ritual.

WHAT YOU DO: Place three strawberries into a bowl of straw and make your wish concerning the following day – either for general luck or financial luck, or for something more specific. Lightly spray some violet-leaf essential oil, diluted with spring water, on to your pillow. Put the bowl of strawberries beside your bed and close your eyes, remembering the pretty image of the nesting strawberries. When you wake in the morning, eat the strawberries one by one, rewording your wish or hopes from the night before accordingly. Take a piece of the straw with you to carry through the day, and give your hair a light spray with some more of the violet-oil-and-spring-water mix. You will be sure to have a very lucky day. This is an excellent wish-spell to do if you have an important interview for a job that you really want. Try it out!

Scented basil wish

If you would like one of your colleagues to notice you as a potential love, or as some-one who is worthy of more money or promotion, make them this special ice cream and serve it for pudding or just in a cone, any time … There is no need for an ice-cream maker, so don't rush out to buy one. Oh, and obviously, a dinner or lunch invi-tation must precede this …

WHAT YOU DO: All the while you are preparing this recipe, repeat: *'I am deserving, and you will notice me.'* Place a vanilla pod in 300 ml (½ pint) double cream in the refrigera-tor, and leave to flavour overnight. The following day, beat three egg yolks with 150 g (5 oz) sugar and stir in six finely chopped basil leaves. Breathe in the scent from them. Whip the cream, and beat the three egg whites until stiff. Using a metal spoon, blend the sugar mixture with the cream and then the whites; finally, add 3 tablespoons sherry. Put the mixture in a mould in the freezer for eight hours. Serve in any easy way, with one fresh basil leaf for presentation.

And then you simply wait to see your impact over the days to follow. Keep a basil plant, or some basil leaves, around your desk or work area for a week or two, and touch the leaves to increase the impact.

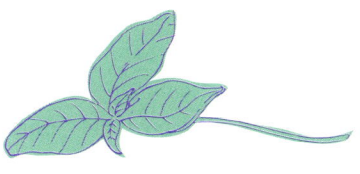

A Prosperous Home: A Ritual for Perpetuity

This ritual is something to do as often as you feel you want to. I still do it twice a year, on the equinoxes, and on occasions I have performed it again on the launch of a new project or work relationship. The aim is to attract beneficence to the home, which is where this should be performed.

This will not make you instantly rich, or even make you become too materialistic in your outlook (don't worry). But it does attract a state of *grace*, I think, so that work relationships are positive, and so that the material world in which we must live is in balance in our lives. There should always be enough food on the plate, and a little over for guests. Perfect prosperity!

YOU WILL NEED: *Diffuser*
Yarrow essential oil
Cubeb oil (mae chang)
Hyssop oil
Music
One peony, or a large scented pink rose if a peony is unavailable (though you should be able to get one from a good florist around the time of the spring equinox)
Special vase or bottle
Scented lilacs, if possible (or lilac perfume oil or violet-leaf essential oil)
Toasted bread

Apple juice (or apple wine – see below)
One small piece of ribbon in white or green satin

WHAT YOU DO: (This must have you wondering!) Choose a day on which to perform this; it need not be the equinox, but could be a birthday, anniversary, 1 May, or any other time to which you are drawn. For the entire day, from sundown till sun-up, and sun-up till sundown again, use your diffuser to scent your home with the aromatic oils listed above. Use about five drops of each in warm water, and recharge as often as is necessary to keep the fragrance going for a full day. At sundown, before the light has gone, put on some elevating music (your choice, but make it something that raises the hairs on your neck!) and place your peony or rose in the vase or bottle. Also, if you can get them, place some fresh lilacs in your bedroom. You need these scents all around your home, inducing a state of grace and joy and abundance and good will towards people. If you can't get lilacs, spray perfume oil or violet-leaf essential oil on to the pillow, as either of these work well too.

Still at sundown, place the toasted bread in apple juice or apple wine. (If you don't have apple wine, but like the idea, you can make some by choosing a dry white wine and infusing it with slices of apples and a light sprinkle of brown sugar for a few hours.) Add some spices to your toast and apple juice if you like. You are making a form of 'wassail' mixture, which you will sip and use to toast your ventures and friends later, so make it palatable! Then take one of the oils used earlier, and dab a little on your ribbon. Take the wine and toast, the ribbon, and the oils in a bottle, out on to your porch or into your garden, or wherever you grow a tree you love. If you are lucky enough to have a big garden, choose three trees (apple was traditional!). Then, still hearing the music (if you are too far away, let it echo in your mind), say: *'I wish and ask a blessing of bounty on all things. May my tree(s), my garden, my friends, my family and my own dreams thrive. May we all prosper in this house.'* Bow to the tree(s) and put a drop or two of oil, and then a special drink of the brew, around the trunk – a cupful is enough. Touch the tree. Tie the ribbon on to one of its branches.

Now come back to your dining or eating area, sip your wine, breathe the medley of scents and listen to the music. Say the words above once more. If you have summoned a real sense of heart and presence of spirit, then the fairylike flowers – peony, rose, lilac – will do all they can to help. You will find an improved sense of luck, prosperity and help with business and finance in the days ahead. And so, do you understand why this ritual is worth repeating?

Fragrant Abundance

The last spell I have chosen is to draw abundance: financial strength, personal productivity and all-round positivity. Abundance can mean love, family and home; it means there is enough – in fact an abundance – of whatever you need. Sounds perfect, really.

YOU WILL NEED: *Fresh herbs*

Three candles, coloured green, white and yellow-gold

5 drops each of bay, frankincense and sandalwood oils

Diffuser

A goblet filled with fresh spring- or rainwater

A crystal (any colour that you are drawn to)

A dark red ribbon

Three flowers (of any colour)

WHAT YOU DO: On a waxing moon, take a bath with fresh herbs added to the water. Bathe by the light of your candles, to the diffused scent of your oils in your burner. Feel the water close to your skin, smell the scents swirling about you, see the light from the candles entering your mind and making it calm and sure. Imagine you are free from debt, though not necessarily rich; free from worry, though not necessarily without positive challenges; and free from negativity at work, though not necessarily lacking tests of your humour sometimes! Balance, and abundance …

Dry yourself, and keep the oils burning. Sit with your goblet, into which you should drop the crystal. Tie the ribbon around the stem of your goblet, take a sip and toast 'abundance', saying: *'I deserve the best things in my life. And so shall it be.'* Then take the crystal and place it with your three flowers near where you sleep or relax (in a lounge or bedroom). Promise quietly to share, and not to have shallow values.

Keep the crystal and flowers together for three days. Every night for three nights, drink something (wine, for instance) from your goblet, still with the ribbon around its stem. On each of these nights, sprinkle a drop of each of the three oils near your front door; on a mat or entry rug is excellent. And every day for the same three days, give one single-stem flower (not one of yours, but a fresh stem) to someone you think needs a smile.

Afterwards, put your crystal in a drawer or place where you keep money or accounts (like a cheque book). This whole spell will draw an incredible power supply to you, and you will find yourself physically 'zinging' for quite some time, and laughing and smiling … abundantly!

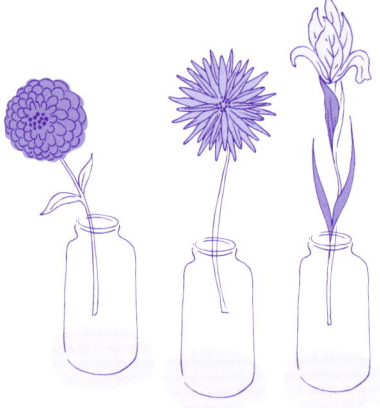

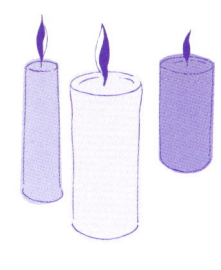

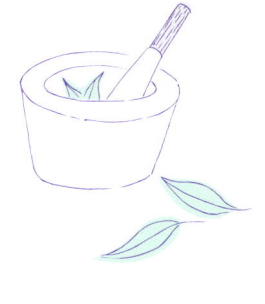

CHAPTER SIX

Healing

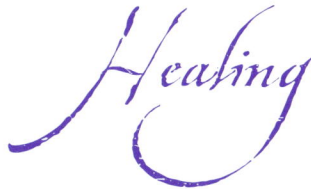

Scent can be used in so many ways during the healing process – not least as a foil to the smells often associated with hospitals or sickrooms. Aromatic herbs and oils heal the ailing spirit as well as the body, which is the most powerful combination for recovery. There are also aromas that counter some common illnesses, or help to speed up the recovery; and if the spirits are under siege, aromatic ritual can help us avoid sliding into illness. So here we explore a few possibilities for prevention, part-cure and recovery. Candles can add something, because the light effects improve the psyche and add strength for battling infection: if your circumstances permit, use a scented candle in place of sprays or diffusers, though in a waiting room or hospital this would not be permitted, of course. Once we can convince the brain to heal the body, we are part of the way there. (PLEASE NOTE: the material in this chapter in no way replaces the diagnosis or treatment of a qualified practitioner. Use the ideas here in tandem, if you like, with professional advice.)

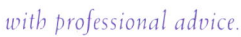

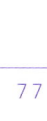

Lifting the Spirits

This is a wonderful ritual to relieve someone who has been ill, depressed, or who is still very run-down after a long bout of illness. It also acts as a relief for the nurses and other people who have been anxious about the patient.

I used this ritual recently when a close friend had suffered a bad burn from scalding tea; the lemon and geranium work both on the shock factor after burns, as well as helping to dispel anxiety. They are also very good in combination for people with bad colds or flu, which depress us and weaken the body.

YOU WILL NEED: *10 drops lemon essential oil*
5 drops geranium essential oil
A spray bottle, such as a perfume atomizer
Spring water
A green ribbon
Soft toy

WHAT YOU DO: Blend the oils in the atomizer with a little spring water – just enough to create a mist. Spritz some of the resulting aromatic mist on to the green ribbon, and on to a soft toy that you will give as a gift to your 'patient'.

A white-coloured toy – such as a baby might hold for softness and size – is ideal, as the white also lifts the spirits and makes the person feel soothed, in a babylike way. As you spritz the toy, imagine sunshine pouring into it, making the toy itself seem somehow 'radiant'. Tie the green ribbon in a bow around the neck of the toy, wishing the patient lightness and removal of pain as you do. Really concentrate in your mind's eye, imagining the person free of pain and worry.

Now you must give the toy to your patient, asking them to breathe in the scent if possible. If you are in a private room or at home, spray some of the mist into the air around the patient; if you are in a hospital, however, you may find it intrusive to others to spray the oils generally. But in either case, spray a little on to the pillows – even if you are in a hospital ward. A little will go a long way and, as you spray, imagine again sunshine penetrating the linen and radiating within the space.

The spell works in several ways: the aromas literally lift the spirits of the sick person, while the toy offers comfort; the green colour emits a powerful healing energy, which helps the mind to neutralize pain. Also, if stroked or held, the soft toy allows the patient to release their own endorphins, those natural 'feel-good' chemical signals that ease pain and make us feel better. Pure magic can also be found in the imagined sunshine and light circling round the patient.

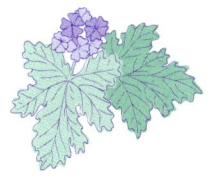

Waging War against Infection

If you have been exposed to a nasty virus, succumbing to the same fate sometimes seems inevitable! But this is not so if you fight the infectious bug aromatically. The oils have antibacterial properties, which make a real physical difference. And our brain has a role to play, too. Not all illnesses are psychosomatic, but our minds can contribute greatly by refusing to believe we will naturally follow suit and become ill. Get out your diffuser, find a very green plant and try waging a war against illness inside the head, and from home!

YOU WILL NEED: *A thriving potted herb with antifungal properties, such as rosemary,*
scented geranium or thyme
10 drops geranium oil
5 drops each eucalyptus and lemon thyme oils
Diffuser
One green ribbon
Lavender or rose geranium soap

WHAT YOU DO: Plant up the herb bush or find one that is already potted, making sure it is healthy and thriving. You will need to caress and play with the leaves, literally stroking them to release the properties of both scent and antiviral powers. Put the herb in the 'hearth' of your home – either a bright kitchen window if you spend a lot of time there, or a well-lit sitting room. Make sure you will come into contact with the plant often. Blend the essential oils into warm water in your diffuser. Burn this fairly frequently over the period that someone is ill around you, and for as long as you need to fight infection yourself. If someone is lingering with a virus that won't give up, this mixture will make an enormous difference to them, and it is very likely to halt the attack on a healthy party altogether.

The other stage of the fight is through the soap and the ribbon. Put one drop of each oil on the ends of the green ribbon and tie it around your head, like a headband, leaving it there for about ten minutes. Do this twice a day. Really imagine the green colour penetrating the corners of your mind, and diffusing just as the oils do through your whole system. Imagine you are a plant absorbing vitality from the colour; imagine you are denying entry to a bug, which you should picture in any way you like. If you do this for a few minutes before bed, it helps the action to kick in while you rest.

And lastly, each morning, wash with the geranium or lavender soap, and envisage the soap sloughing away the feelings of illness, tiredness or being run-down that you might have been victim to. I keep a loofah-quality soap with 'bits in', as my daughter says, just for this purpose – to scour off gently any accretions of illness that might come from the outside world.

If you keep up this three-pronged attack – oils and herb, ribbon around the mind, and showering – for a few days, you will not only keep gremlins at bay, but should also experience a fantastic feeling of well-being and increased vitality. We should all do it once a month, to charge our batteries and shed the dross the world throws at us in traffic and closed environments. Nearly as good as a holiday!

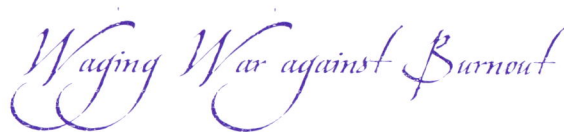

Waging War against Burnout

Before you become ill, try this calming and fortifying ritual to help ease back the nerves and get your mind, body and spirit flowing happily together.

There is much we can do to stop ourselves succumbing to illness when we know we are functioning near to burnout. Perhaps we have too much emotional matter to deal with, coupled with overwork and feelings of panic about how much we have to get through? Maybe all of our inner reserves have been depleted? So often we endure an intense moment when several woes seem to fall in a heap together. But fear not – help is at hand …

YOU WILL NEED: *One gardenia flower (often available throughout the year in cool climates, where they must be kept indoors)*
Glass bowl
Rose, jasmine or verbena tea
A blend of four oils in total (3 drops each) from lemon balm, lemon grass or lemon verbena with lemon, marjoram and vetiver
Diffuser

WHAT YOU DO: This is a soothing ritual and it is worth doing it properly, even if it sounds a little odd. The mind must work in tandem with the body, as burnout is both physical and emotional. So, sit near an open window, and take three long breaths of regular rhythm. Hum gently on any note that is comfortable for you to reach. Hum

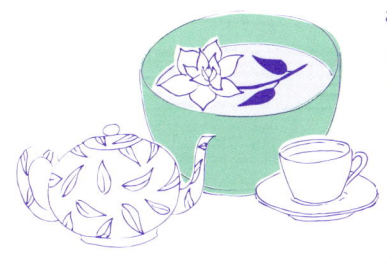

a melody you like, or just hum a nice, resonating single note. Now put the gardenia flower (nothing else is quite as good, but a white hyacinth or orange blossom would be a good second choice if you really can't find a gardenia) in warm water, in the glass bowl, where you can really enjoy the prettiness of the flower. Inhale the scent deeply. Take in the colour white and imagine it entering right into your soul until you can feel your chest give a little upward 'tug' – you will know what this is as soon as you experience it. Rest on that uplifting note for a second and feel the light coursing through you, chasing away tiredness and melancholy. It is important to say something to yourself like: *'Life is a mixture of joys and sorrows, stresses and pleasures – but I would not be anywhere else other than "in" it!'* Close your eyes, feel the light, the fresh air and the scent of the flower.

Now make up your tea, and sip it slowly, while you diffuse the oils in your burner for exactly half an hour. Do this in a quiet moment towards the close of the day, perhaps before bed. And if you indulge yourself with this ritual three or more times over a week, your spirits will lift and the weight will seem to lift, permitting you to deal with the burdens and at the same time avoid real burnout. Do this as often as you need to – the effect seems almost cumulative.

Anxiety Relief

This little ritual helps when someone close to you is ill, or perhaps undergoing an operation. They will borrow your strength, so make sure you have some to offer.

When you are anxiously waiting on someone's results, a birth or for an operation to finish, this will help give you back the strength that you will need to support the patient.

YOU WILL NEED: *Bach Rescue Remedy*
100 ml (4 fl oz) spring water
10 drops each geranium and lemon
essential oils
A spray bottle (or perfume atomizer)
A small, decorative tree branch (if it is
spring, blossom would be wonderful, but
any pretty, small branch will work wonders)
One yellow and one green ribbon

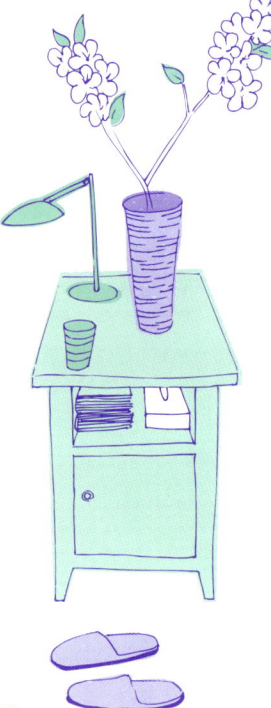

WHAT YOU DO: When you are anxiously waiting on something beyond your control, always use Rescue Remedy, as it relieves the stress of being inactive. Then, if you are in a hospital waiting room, mix up a spring-water spray with the water and essential oils. Shake the bottle and spray into a general area that will not interfere with others; if this is impossible, spray it near your own head – even very lightly around your face (after closing your eyes). This combination has a wonderful impact when you are running on exhaustion, for the lemon revives while the geranium relieves. Use the spray to mist lightly near the patient during recovery, as well (unless it is a young child or baby – in which case, only mild lavender oil is permitted).

Place the branch near the patient and tie the two coloured ribbons around it. The colour and the power of the tree spirit work to relieve the anxious feelings and calm the spirit to quiet anticipation of a better result. They also speed the healing of the patient. Nothing seems to work better than the green of trees. In the same way, if you have the opportunity, wait for news in a garden, rather than inside a more sterile environment such as a hospital or clinic.

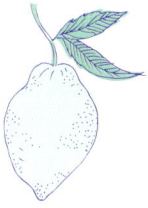

To Reduce Tiredness and Nausea in Pregnancy

When you are pregnant your whole system is under siege, although it seems to thrive, so it is essential to get those feet up and take time to treat yourself. This charm is chosen carefully, with a mild infusion of safe oils for use in pregnancy. Do it when you are overwrought, tired or want some healthy pampering.

YOU WILL NEED: *2 drops each camomile, lavender and geranium oils* (ONLY THESE THREE!)
Diffuser
Satin or silken socks (or slippers)
A few mildly scented rose petals
Silk pillow slip or cloth

WHAT YOU DO: When you are feeling weary, diffuse the oils somewhere you can lie down. Put on the tactile socks – the tactility is vital, as it helps to release your body's endorphins, the feel-good chemicals. Lie back and scatter a few rose petals at your head: rose signals to our system that we are at peace, which helps to convince your placenta to stop making you feel so ill, as you are both on the same side! The silky pillow slip, or cloth over the pillow, caresses your head, hair and neck and releases your endorphins (which also naturally counter some of the aches and pains). Rub your temples a little, and send pink loving thoughts to your bump and your placenta. Tell them you love and accept them, however different they are from you! Finally, close your eyes, allowing the aromas to penetrate for a good fifteen minutes. Don't hurry. When you re-emerge into the 'real' world, you will feel as though you've had at least two hours' sleep!

To Caress Someone Who is Ill

The tree comes into its own again in this powerful ritual. Other elements will help whenever you have to care for someone who is convalescing, or really in the thick of illness.

WHAT YOU DO: As for the *Anxiety Relief* ritual on page 84, take a blossoming tree branch, but this time put a photo of the person who is ill (showing them when they were in better health) among the foliage. Every day, spray the tree lightly with a mist of diluted oils in 100 ml (4 fl oz) spring water: if the patient is male, use 5 drops each coriander, mandarin and scented geranium oils; if the patient is female, use myrrh, melissa (lemon balm) and geranium. Of course, the tree branch should be near enough for the convalescent also to benefit from the scents.

It is also important that twice a day you stroke the person being cared for on their hands – using hand cream if possible. A lemon-based cream will help to lend them more energy to recover.

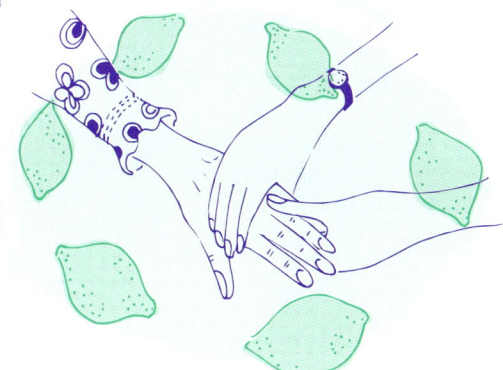

To Nurse Someone in Their Own Home

Once a patient has returned home, the best healers are natural herbs – in a basket,
or among the patient's personal items.

WHAT YOU DO: Make up a window box or a hanging basket, where the patient can both see and smell the collection of scented herbs. Use lemon-scented plants like thyme and verbena or lemon balm, as well as soft mauve-flowering plants such as catmint, lavender, santolina and violets. Each time you walk past, touch them with your fingertips to release the scent; if possible, get your patient to do this, too.

Also, treat your patient to a new pretty pair of slippers, into which you should place muslin bags scented with herbs: lavender, peppermint and geranium leaves are nearly always the best choice for healing. The feet are very important when we are sick; relief for them can help heal in myriad ways. Encourage them to wear the little slippers each time they walk around, and to put back the scented bags when they are not being used, to allow the scent to recharge. You could also make up a muslin bag, trimmed with pale green ribbon, to slip over the coat hanger on which the patient's dressing robe or bed-cardigan hangs. Use the same scents, plus anything lemon-scented. A bag like this could be taken into a hospital as well, to cheer a patient while they are there. These herbs can really help someone who is ill to find the energy and courage to fight their condition. The ritual may not work miracles outright, but it will lend an enormous amount of help, and also make you feel you as though you have been able to offer them a little natural, aromatic support.

Appendix

A quick-reference chart to the oils

This quick-reference chart gives you an overview of some of the main oils we have used, and suggests their most important associations so that you can use them – at a glance – in any situation. Many oils offer similar benefits, so feel free to substitute if an oil you have does similar things to one you don't. This list is by no means exhaustive, and if you want to take it further there are some suggestions for further reading on page 94.

AROMA OIL	ASSOCIATION	FOR
Basil	*Stimulating*	Memory, positivity, cheerfulness, clarity, concentration, energy, cleanliness, reducing fatigue, removing indecisiveness
Benzoin	*Well-being*	Easing anxiety, healing, soothing, inner quiet, peace
Bergamot	*Refreshing*	Motivation, uplifting feeling, hope, confidence, positivity, reducing depression, calming anxiety, feeling renewed
Cardamom	*Enthusing*	Courage, strength, improved concentration, more tolerance, endurance, battling apathy
Carnation	*Sensual*	Communication, feeling freer, dealing with criticism, countering loneliness, feeling poised, thinking deeply
Cedarwood	*Emboldening*	Greater stability, dealing with worry, focusing, exuding dignity, feet on the ground, dispelling gloom, countering doubts
(Roman) Camomile	*Soothing*	Peace, relaxation, healing, soothing when tender, countering nerves, patience, calming a temper, managing a crisis; also suitable to use during pregnancy in mild, diluted forms (massage, bath, mild diffusion)
Moroccan Camomile (also called Ormenis Flower)		Feeling spiritual, unwinding, releasing problems/stress, slowing down, dealing with temper, reducing nervousness and fears
Cinnamon	*Heartening*	Feeling warm, being practical, greater energy, awareness of others, even-temper, countering moodiness, rationality

AROMA OIL	ASSOCIATION	FOR
Coriander	*Motivating*	Imagination, reasoning power, memory, confidence, moodiness, buoyancy, enthusiasm, countering stress
Cubeb (mae chang)		Wisdom and confidence
Cypress	*Noble*	Healing, energizing, clarifying, fighting viruses, stability, confidence, willpower, fuller understanding, fair-mindedness
Eucalyptus	*Emboldening, balancing*	Antiviral, antifungal, cheerfulness, exuberance, reducing moodiness, calming a frayed temper, rational thinking, energy, certainty
Frankincense	*Spirit-giving*	Meditation, calmness, higher wisdom, self-belief, enlightened thought, inspiration, loving to mankind, healing, dispelling despair
Gardenia (likely to be found as an absolu or fragrance oil – expensive, so dilute)	*Soulful, exotic*	Warmth, sensuality, femininity, brightness of mind, calming headaches, soothing nerves, countering bad temper, being 'in touch', sensitivity, dreaminess
Scented Geranium	*Uplifting*	Tonic effect, calming nerves, wisdom, kindness, coping, flexibility, feeling secure, inducing tranquillity, calming fears, feeling loving, being responsive, soothing in crises, reducing confusion, high-minded, humour; in pregnancy, as with camomile and lavender, can be safely used in very mild form
Ginger	*Energizing, encouraging*	Alertness, sympathetic feeling, warmth, focus, gentle vigour, battling burnout, feeling refreshed, sensuality
Grapefruit	*Blossoming*	Opening up, feeling joy, experiencing things to the full, waking, encouraging, laughter, battling apathy, countering frustrations, feeling creative
Hyacinth	*Flirtatious*	Gentleness, good humour, positivity, creativity, good self-feeling, tolerance to others, calming sadness, fighting emotional heartache
Hyssop	*Industriousness*	Overwork, depression, alertness, dealing with grief or guilt, good oil for working smoothly and well, lucky!

AROMA OIL	ASSOCIATION	FOR
Immortelle (also called Italian Everlasting and Helichrysum)		Cosmetic use, uplift, clarity with gentleness, idealism, productivity, good dreams, soothing overwork, handling bad news, coping with change, inner calm, self-confidence
Jasmine	*Erotic*	Everything(!), including sensuality, more energy, confidence, relaxation, inspiration, harmony, countering self-doubts, joyfulness, hospitality, countering emotional crises and worries; use diluted for massage during birth process
Juniper	*Radiant*	Cleansing feeling, wisdom, profound thoughts, creativity
Lavender	*Calming*	Also, everything – a must-have for the oil cabinet! – including security, calming nerves and exhaustion, keeping alert but relaxed, preventing burnout, compassion, vitality, feeling younger, countering sadness and moods, peace and balance, feeling childlike, dealing with irritability; antibacterial, good for burns and skin complaints, can be used neat and also safe for mild use throughout pregnancy
Lemon	*Boosting*	Awareness, concentration, hope, energy, humour, clarity, confidence, memory, trauma; good neat on spots, mosquito bites, etc.
Lemon Balm (Melissa)	*Supporting*	Women, vitality, liveliness, warm-heartedness, countering anxiety and emotional frigidity, cheerfulness, sensibility, kindness, progressive thinking, strength, relaxation
Lemon Thyme		*as Thyme*
Lemon Verbena (hard to get as an essential oil, but use in body lotions and bath products)	*Lightening*	As an absolu, lifts spirits, helps to cope with confusion, lessens insomnia, feels 'clean'
Mandarin	*Gentleness*	Energy, hope, charisma, kindness, good humour, letting go, child-like qualities, reducing grief, sensuality, sympathy
Marjoram	*Joyousness*	Warmth, cheer, assurance, inner calm, inner knowing, reducing irrational doubts, healing, pleasures
Myrrh	*High-mindedness*	Sensuality, nobility, inspiration, clearing the mind

AROMA OIL	ASSOCIATION	FOR
Narcissus	*Hypnotic*	Sensuality, dreaminess, ideas, courage, passion, visions, creativity, battling hopelessness and dejection, boosting self-image, treating shock
Neroli (expensive, but worth it – a must-have oil)	*Purity, spirituality*	Love, happiness, gentle confidence, satisfaction, lifting sadness or stress, countering fatigue, loss of sensuality, feeling flirty and light-hearted, expressive, complete, optimism, against grief or fear; use in marriage ceremonies and birthing process
Orange	*Energy, spark*	Sunshine demeanour, exuding happiness, feeling strong and courageous, sympathy to others, good determination, against emotional bullying
Oregano		*as Marjoram*
Patchouli	*Stability*	Feeling on top, taking control, meditative qualities, happiness, astute ideas, perceptiveness, combating lethargy or apathy, regenerative
Peony (find as an absolu or perfume oil, which is worth the search)	*Abundance*	Feeling lucky, light-hearted, prosperous, sweet-natured, believing in goodness of life, hospitality, exoticism, originality, countering laziness or feeling drab
Peppermint	*Wide awake*	Clarity, confidence, memory, energy, vibrancy, combating overwork, getting engine moving
Petigrain	*Restorative*	Strength and focus, confidence, ability to talk, reducing sleeplessness, combating sadness or anger, balancing moods
Pine	*Cleansing*	Brightness, healing against coughs and colds, good spirit, warming in winter, feeling for others, forgiving, trusting, humble feelings
Rose Maroc (Rosa centifolia)	*Bliss!*	Sensuality, femininity, passion, humanity, open to love, feeling free, counters frigidity or loss of sexual confidence, motivates, soothes jealousy and nervousness, soothes, harmonizes, warms, good for sleep

AROMA OIL	ASSOCIATION	FOR
Rose Otto *(Rosa damascena)* (expensive, so buy an absolu if need be, but the most all-reducing round performer of all the oils – a must-have)	*Euphoria*	Everything, including love, care of others, good heart, good cheer, self-awareness, self-understanding, forgiveness, calm, sensuality, devotion, comfort, wisdom, patience, motivation, revival, renewal, joy, pleasure, good skin, self-worth, reducing addictive behaviour, consoling emotional hurts, aiding in a crisis, assisting parents, brightening and soothing children
Rosemary	*Focusing*	Memory, positivity, male sexuality, fighting exhaustion
Sandalwood	*Enlightening*	Noble thoughts, courage, spiritual feelings, surviving stress or insults, creating harmony, bringing serenity, calming – especially men
Tea Tree (no Australian home would be without it)	*Vividness*	The most powerful known antiseptic, it is antifungal, antiviral, treats skin sores and wounds, bites; also boosts energy, confidence, immune system, vibrancy, self-control, self-belief, counters fatigue, hypochondria and loss of youthful feelings
Thyme	*Supportive*	Antibacterial properties, alertness, tolerance, making decisions, cleansing environment, letting go of the past
Tuberose (my other favourite with gardenia and rose)	*Extrovert*	Aiding free expression, sensuality, self-image, laughter, enigmatic qualities, enthusiasm, sensitivity, creativity, fighting stress and disorientation, soothing hostility/selfishness
Vetiver (my husband's favourite!)	*Visionary*	Bestowing kindness, patience, integrity, feelings of honour, human fellow feeling, countering exhaustion, overwork and emotional damage from the past, soothing nervous behaviour, reducing anger
Violet (Leaf) (experiment with it!)	*Romantic*	Elfin qualities – loving, uplifting, extraordinary; use also in cosmetic preparations
Yarrow	*Contemplative*	Meditation, healing, handling sorrow, business focus
Ylang Ylang	*Elevating*	Emotional warmth, joy, combating resentment and arrogance, countering stubbornness and jealousies

Further Reading

This subject is inexhaustible, and there are a great many good books on the subject of aromatherapy. Some of my favourites are listed below.

Aromantics, Valerie A. Worwood, Bantam Books, 1987.

The Fragrant Herbal, Lesley Bremness, Quadrille, 1998. (This details many beautiful ways to employ herbs for scent, and also offers excellent information on oils.)

The Fragrant Pharmacy, Valerie A. Worwood, Bantam Books, 1990. (Both this and the previous volume by Worwood are essential reading, together forming a virtual bible from the leading name in the business.)

The Herb Society's Complete Medicinal Herbal, Penelope Ody, Dorling Kindersley, 1993. (This is a brilliant analysis of the properties of herbs and flowers, the oils, and some other ways to extract their aromas.)

Suppliers

Bach Flower Therapy
Mount Vernon, Sotwell, Wallingford, Oxfordshire, OX10 UK
T: +44 (0)1491 834678
Makers of rescue remedy and other flower essences

Butterbur & Sage
Head Office, Aroma House, 7 Tessa Road, Reading, RG1 8HH UK
T: +44 (0)118 9505100
www.butterburandsage.com
Stock high quality oils, essences and absolutes

The Essential Oil Company
Portland, Oregon USA
www.essentialoil.com
Carry gardenia, frangipani, carnation and peony perfume oils, as well as tuberose absolute

Essentially Yours
P.O. Box 6069, Long Beach, CA 90806 USA
T: +1 (562) 599 5558
email: info@essyrs.com
www.essyrs.com
Offer therapeutic grade oils

Hartwood Aromatics

Enterprise House, Courtaulds Way, Coventry,
West Midlands, CV6 5NX UK
T: +44 (0)2476 667071
Stock a variety of essential oils and essences

Holland & Barrett

Stores throughout the UK, plus catalogue for
mail order and Internet shopping.
www.hollandandbarrett.co.uk
For catalogues and mail order, tel: 0870 606
6606; email: hbcustsrv@hollandandbarrett.com.
For product information and enquiries, email:
Healthinformation@hollandandbarrett.com
Stock a great many oils including gingko essence

Maitre Parfumier et Gantier

Paris, France
Tel: +33 45 44 61 57
*Offer tuberose (which they call Fleurs blanches),
by mail order if you cannot find it elsewhere*

Neal's Yard Remedies

Shops and therapy rooms around the UK, plus
mail order and Internet shopping. Products also
available in the USA and Japan.
Head Office, 8–10 Ingate Place, Battersea,
London, SW8 3NS UK
T: +44 (0)20 7498 1686
F: +44 (0)20 7498 2505
email: mail@nealsyardremedies.com
www.nealsyardremedies.com
www.nealsyardremediesusa.com
For mail order call: 0845 262 3145

*Offer oils, flower essences and damiana and
gingko essences*

SPACE.NK

Stores, spas and stockists around the UK, plus
mail order.
For enquiries please contact the head office:
SPACE.NK Ltd, 200 Great Portland Street,
London, W1W 5QG UK
T: +44 (0)20 7299 4999
www.spacenk.com
Mail order: +44 (0)20 7727 8002
*Stock an unscented pheromone called 'Falling
in Love' by Philosophy*

Star Child

Glastonbury, UK
www.starchild.co.uk
www.starchild-international.com
sales@starchild-international.com
*Offer many products including oils (including
tuberose), organic herbs, flower waters and
tree oils*

Sweet Cakes Soaps

Minnesota, USA
T: +1 (952) 945 9900
Fax: +1 (952) 945-9905
email: info@sweetcakes.com
www.sweetcakes.com
*Carries gardenia and peony fragrance oils (quite
a find) and offer mail order*

About the Author

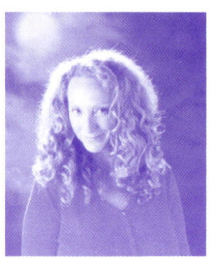

TITANIA HARDIE is Britain's most famous White Witch. Through her mother's guidance she nurtured her own psychic abilities and developed a deep affinity for understanding nature and harnessing its power to enhance lives and well-being. Titania has a degree in psychology and has trained in para-psychology and horary astrology. She also has degrees in English literature and romantic studies. She has made hundreds of television appearances around the world, and has received widespread national newspaper and magazine coverage.

Her previous titles include *Hocus Pocus, Titania's Fortune Cards*, *Dreamtime* and *Titania's Crystal Ball*. In 2002, Boots the Chemist (UK) successfully launched Titania Hardie Beauty Spells, an exclusive collection of magic and bath and beauty products.

Acknowledgements

Scented bouquets to Ian Jackson, Elaine Partington and all the team at Eddison Sadd, and to my wonderful daughters.

Author photograph by Sara Morris.

EDDISON•SADD EDITIONS
EDITORIAL DIRECTOR Ian Jackson
PROJECT EDITORS Katie Ginn and Tessa Monina
COPY-EDITOR Nicki Marshall
PROOFREADER Nikky Twyman
ART DIRECTOR Elaine Partington
MAC DESIGNER Malcolm Smythe
PRODUCTION Sarah Rooney and Nick Eddison